Total Quality in
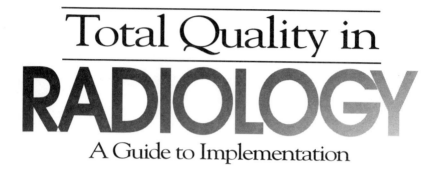
RADIOLOGY
A Guide to Implementation

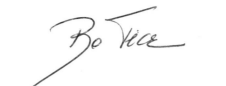

Total Quality in

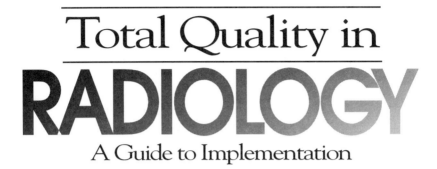

A Guide to Implementation

Authors

Henry George Adams, M.D.
Chairman, Department of Radiology
Lakewood Hospital
Lakewood, Ohio

Sudhir Arora, M.D.
Assistant Professor of Radiology and Nuclear Medicine
Uniformed Services University of Health Sciences
Department of Radiology
National Naval Medical Center
Senior Consultant, National Institutes of Health
Bethesda, Maryland

Copublished by
St. Lucie Press
and the
American Healthcare Radiology Administrators Education Foundation
through an
Educational Grant from Berlex Laboratories

S^{t}L

Library of Congress Cataloging-in-Publication Data

Adams, Henry George, 1947–
    Total quality in radiology : a guide to implementation / by Henry George Adams, Sudhir Arora.
        p.   cm.
    Includes bibliographical references and index.
    ISBN 1-884015-07-7 : $39.95
        1. Hospitals—Radiological services—Administration.
    2. Hospitals—Radiological services—Quality control. 3. Total quality management. 4. Radiology, Medical—Quality control.
    I. Arora, Sudhir, 1951–   II. Title.
        [DNLM: 1. Radiology—organization & administration. 2. Quality Control. WN 100 A213t 1993]
    RA975.5.R3A33   1993
    362.1'77—dc20
DNLM/DLC
for Library of Congress   93-41954
                                                                                       CIP

    Direct all inquiries to St. Lucie Press, Inc., 100 E. Linton Blvd., Suite 403B, Delray Beach, Florida 33483.
    Phone: (407) 274-9906
    Fax: (407) 274-9927   SL^t

Published by
St. Lucie Press
100 E. Linton Blvd., Suite 403B
Delray Beach, FL 33483

DEDICATION

To those who contributed to the new management tools and philosophies: Dr. W. A. Sherwart, Dr. W. R. Deming, Dr. K. Ishikawa, Dr. J. M. Juran, Dr. P. B. Crosby, and to all those workers, past, present, and future, whose expertise will carry the new philosophy toward an ever improving healthcare system, this book is humbly dedicated.

ACKNOWLEDGMENTS

There are many to acknowledge for their understanding, contributions, and encouragements during the conception of this idea and the long hours of drafting and editing text. To the many "willing workers" that made the effort of TQM worthwhile and educated us in the process, to Admiral Donald F. Hagan, currently Surgeon General of the Navy, who inspired us to take up the mantle of change and gave us the courage to try something new and necessary, to Captain Mary Ann Arnold, MC, USN (Retired) for the caring manner in which she taught quality in the medical setting, to Steven E. Liston, M.D., FACR, a mentor and respected member of the profession for his leadership, to Captain David Snyder, MC, USN who knows TQM better than any physician I know and had the wisdom to let us learn it in a way that would work for us, to Mr. Fred DeGrandis, President, Saint John Westshore Hospital, who gave us the opportunity to introduce TQM in a community hospital setting, to Mr. William Baiocchi, Chief Operating Officer of Lakewood Hospital, whose guidance and tolerance allowed TQM to move forward, to the Board of Trustees and Mr. Jules Bouthillet, Chief Executive Officer, Lakewood Hospital, who allowed us to try it, to Mr. David Denecke, Director of Quality, Philips Medical Systems for his advice in reviewing the text, and to Mr. Dennis Buda, Ms. Sandy Pearlman, and Ms. Mary Beth Ross at St. Lucie Press, we owe a sincere debt of gratitude.

To our families LuAnn, Elyse, Lauren, Kamni, Samir, and Reshma, who went without the attention they deserved on the many occasions writing and editing took priority after returning home from our full time jobs, we owe the most thanks for their support and perseverance during the production of this book.

CONTENTS

AUTHOR PREFACE

The idea for this book was conceived while we wrestled new paradigms of management and the difficulty of how to begin the process of empowering those who had long been oppressed with our ineffective management styles. We discovered that implementation is a process just as manufacturing and service. As leaders in this venture, we served in the beginning as the suppliers, providing the input and taking action to provide a desired output to those who were out there doing their best every day, in many cases without the proper tools.

We also discovered that satisfying the customer is more important than we ever believed before and that the customer within our organization is as important as the one receiving our product.

In our walk with Total Quality we also discovered there was no one source of information which facilitates the learning and understanding of TQM. Also, examples of implementation and experience were non-existent. With this book we hope we have corrected this deficiency.

Reading this book will not make your radiology department better but it may make you a better manager and/or radiologist. It will give you the basic tools to begin the process of change toward continuous improvement so that you can lead the improvement of your organization.

It is not a panacea or remedy for health care reform but a preventive program against failure with a purpose of promoting continued success in the face of difficult times. In these times of remarkable change our best weapon of defense is knowledge and proof of what is in the best interests of good patient care. The analysis derived from the tools of TQM can yield us the knowledge needed to combat naive proposals that may harm the public good.

Our fervent wish is that this book rekindles that fire of excellence we all had when we began our professional careers, nurtures the notion that we can make a difference in health care outcomes, and most of all we hope our patients all benefit from it.

Henry George Adams, M.D.
Sudhir Arora, M.D.

Part I

THE BASICS

1

INTRODUCTION to TOTAL QUALITY MANAGEMENT

INTRODUCTION

Is the practice of radiology in the United States heading toward a state of crisis? Do external influences threaten to remove the autonomy of the practice enjoyed since the discovery of the X-ray? Is the economic structure of today's practice changing unfavorably? Are inroads in the practice of radiology being made by individuals not trained in diagnosis? Many would respond affirmatively, but why?

Healthcare cost currently represents about 13% of the Gross Domestic Product (GDP) in the United States, which is the highest percentage among the five other major industrialized countries. If the cost continues to escalate at the present rate, by the turn of the century it may be 16 to 20% of the GDP. What do we have to show for this? Despite an inordinate financial outlay, the infant mortality rate in the United States is the highest compared to the same five countries. We do not even rank among the top ten countries with the lowest infant mortality rate. In addition, over 37 million Americans are either uninsured or underinsured for healthcare. The high cost of healthcare, which some measure as the most expensive per capita in the world, certainly harms the poor and underinsured. In addition, it has the potential to hinder the success of businesses which drive this economy in the world marketplace.

The American healthcare consumer is becoming much more intelligent and informed regarding his or her care and is demanding more for the expense. Public confidence in leaders of organized medicine has fallen from 73% in the mid-1960s to 33% in 1986. The vast majority of Americans believe that the increased cost of healthcare is not justified, and they believe that rising costs can be reduced by better organization and management, without cutting the quality of care. Failing that, there

3

is rising public interest in mandated controls on costs. This interest is being transmitted to public policymakers who affect government-subsidized healthcare programs.

Cost and quality control mandates are already in place for radiologists as a result of the public perception of poor quality. The Breast and Cervical Cancer Screening Mortality Prevention Act of 1990 is the direct result of the public outcry for improved quality. This act mandates certain standards in mammography and Pap smear screening. The Breast Cancer Quality Improvement Act of 1992 requires all mammography sites to be certified.

Some states (Michigan, New Mexico) have already passed laws requiring certain standards for mammography screening. In others (Kentucky, District of Columbia), insurers require accreditation before payment of mammography fees.

Whether or not this can be considered misdirected control of costs, physician reimbursements are coming under more intense downward pressure under the Resource Based Relative Value Scale (RBRVS) in an effort to reduce costs without concern for quality. One can only interpret from this that the future of radiologic practice, where radiologists are told not only how much they will be paid for their work but also how they are to accomplish it, is here today.

Highly advanced technology has proliferated throughout the healthcare system and added to the cost of care, sometimes without benefit in the outcome of a patient encounter. Some find this state-of-the-art technology unnecessary; others demand it as a sign that they are receiving "quality" care. Excessive malpractice suits and awards have fueled overutilization of these diagnostic technologies.

The financial health of healthcare institutions is also of concern. Nearly 700 hospitals in the United States went out of business in the 1980s. Reasons for these closures include reduced federal reimbursements for Medicaid and Medicare patients, the high cost of emergency trauma care, caring for uninsured patients who are unable to pay, and in some cases a shortage of healthcare workers. This is convincing evidence that the U.S. healthcare system, and along with it radiology and its high-cost imaging procedures, is in crisis.

Fundamental changes are needed in the ways the healthcare industry conducts business. Tort reform is not the only answer. Adjudicated and legislated policies are not an acceptable answer. The best defense for the healthcare profession is a good offense. As providers, we can apply our scientific skills and leadership to improve the medical knowledge base and provide a better product. As administrators, we can apply new management skills to root out problems in productivity, improve satisfaction of our customers, and better serve the needs of our patients. These answers imply a return to the basics of the industry: the needs of patients and the quality of care.

Total Quality Management (TQM), which focuses on the needs and expectations of customers and the continuous improvement of the product, applies as well to radiology as it has to many Fortune 500 industries. By adopting the principles of TQM, other industrial organizations have reduced operating expenses while improving consumer satisfaction and company profitability. To survive in the decades ahead, the healthcare industry, and radiology along with it, can build upon the valuable experience gained by other service industries: improved quality leads to improved productivity, which leads to greater market share.

A wide variety of terms have been used for quality management, including Total Quality Management (TQM), Total Quality Control (TQC), Total Quality Leadership (TQL), Total Quality Improvement (TQI), Statistical Quality Control (SQC), and Continuous Quality Improvement (CQI). The term is less significant than the substance. The intent is the same: to improve the product and increase market share.

TQM is a structured, systematic approach in which all employees are utilized as a source of ideas in order to continuously improve processes, services, and products. The system integrates the development, maintenance, and improvement of quality in a never-ending cycle to produce a product or service that satisfies the customer's needs and expectations.

The quality of any product can be gauged by multiple objective criteria, such as durability, conformance to standards, reliability, performance, and serviceability. The quality of a service is perceived by the customer and is often measured against customer expectations. Because expectations (what is acceptable) are always changing, the system mandates continual awareness of customer needs and requirements and implementation of appropriate action; hence, the term continuous improvement.

TQM is based on the following premises:

- Due to their intimate knowledge of job conditions, those workers closest to the problem are more likely to know what is wrong with a process and how to fix it.
- Every person in the organization wants to be a valuable contributor and wants to do a good job.
- Such contributions provide the employee a sense of ownership and reduce adversarial relationships between workers and management.

- Processes, not people, are the root of quality problems. The system is the cause of the problem 85% of the time; the cause is personnel 15% of the time (the 85/15 rule).
- A structured problem-solving process using statistical means produces better long-term solutions than an unstructured process.
- Quality improvement is everyone's job because all processes can be improved; in healthcare, all processes are interrelated by one common factor: the patient.
- Practicing in an environment of fear is counterproductive and leads to poor performance in the long run.
- 80% of the problems are the result of 20% of the causes (the 80/20 rule).

This book goes beyond methods for ensuring quality. Meeting standards is no longer sufficient to stay in business. We must move beyond measuring quality and toward improving it—continuously. It is our intention to introduce the radiologist and radiology administrator to the fundamentals of TQM, present the basic tools of TQM as they apply to the practice of diagnostic radiology, and demonstrate how simple statistical methods with a focus on improving processes can transform a radiologic practice with long-standing frustrations into a business with long-term rewards.

HISTORICAL PERSPECTIVE

The need for quality products and services has existed since the beginning of civilization. Prior to the Industrial Revolution, however, quality controls were implemented either by consumer inspection of goods or by the artisan's concept of what the consumer wants and the desire to maintain his reputation. The Industrial Revolution led to greater production output, which mandated implementing quality inspection to ensure adherence to specifications for materials, process, and finished goods.

In the late 19th century, Frederick Winslow Taylor formulated a system of "Scientific Management." According to Taylor's system, specialists formulated technical and work standards and required workers to follow these specifications. Although this system led to a considerable increase in productivity, it resulted in stagnation of quality improvement. The system was based on the premise that the worker is unmotivated and needs a system of controls and continual direction. It did not take into account worker potential and the desire to contribute.

Dr. W. A. Shewhart from Bell Laboratories is credited with the inception of quality control as we know it today. Among other contributions, in the late 1930s he created the control chart, which was put to use during the Second World War and was instrumental in the United States being able to produce massive quantities of reliable, state-of-the-art military equipment economically. After the war, when the United States was the only major industrialized nation that could produce the goods that the remainder of the recovering world needed, American production management began to focus on quantity rather than quality. Increased quality was equated with decreased productivity, and the standard became the least acceptable quality to market a product. Depending on individual perspective, this attitude may or may not have found its way into medicine during this period of time.

Total quality control was introduced in Japan in 1946 by U.S. occupation forces. To overcome the unreliability of the Japanese telephone system, the former Bell Labs engineers on General Douglas MacArthur's staff transplanted the American method of quality control to the Japanese telecommunication industry. Despite early problems, the method produced promising results and was adopted by other Japanese industries. In addition, in 1950 General MacArthur invited Dr. W. Edwards Deming to Japan to conduct a population census. During his visits, Deming gave a series of lectures on statistical quality control to top business and academic leaders, providing advice on the importance of recognizing dispersion in statistics, the use of control charts for process control, and the use of the plan, do, check, act (PDCA) cycle (known in Japan as the Deming cycle but actually an adaptation of the Shewhart cycle).

Dr. J. M. Juran's visit to Japan in 1954 helped convince Japanese business leaders to consider quality control as a management tool and started the total quality control movement. The results speak for themselves. The remarkable shift in perception of products "made in Japan" from the early 1960s to the present is testimony enough.

Deming's and Juran's principles were reintroduced in the United States after a quarter century of demonstrable quality improvement in Japanese industry. In the 1980s, TQM was successfully implemented by many Fortune 500 companies in the United States. The earliest American implementation of TQM was in the manufacturing industry, but more recently the techniques have been successfully translated into such service industries such as finance, hotels, and healthcare.

QUALITY ASSURANCE vs. QUALITY IMPROVEMENT

Figures like this tell the management how things have been going, but they do not point the way to improvement.

W. Edwards Deming

Defining quality in healthcare is not an easy task. Many have devoted considerable effort in that regard and yet little agreement exists as to what constitutes quality in healthcare. Some define it as the success of a procedure or the result of therapeutics. Many patients, however, have been dissatisfied with their care because they felt mistreated personally. The organization that touts the training and skill of its radiologists will still experience difficulties if patients are not satisfied with how they are treated during the encounter.

TQM embraces the concept of improving quality, rather than assuring it. It is frequently said that quality cannot be assured—it must be built in. Those organizations that continue to just meet standards will soon fall behind those that meet new improved standards of care. In a competitive marketplace, the former will not be in business for long in the coming healthcare environment.

The implementation of Quality Assurance (QA) in the healthcare industry over the past decade was an important step in reinforcing standards of care, where standards had previously been loosely applied. Unfortunately, the focus of QA was on the individual provider as the source of poor outcomes (the bad apple theory).

Despite this obvious shortcoming, there were some positive aspects. Attention was directed toward high-priority clinical care (high volume, high cost, and problem prone), toward the development and use of relevant clinical indicators, and toward the analysis of appropriate and effective care.

However, interrelated governance, managerial, and support processes were virtually ignored, leaving the practitioner solely accountable for actions over which he or she had little control. Action was frequently initiated only after a problem was identified, and no recognition was given to the difference between "doing things right" and "doing the right thing," a problem in standards-driven systems.

As an example, in QA the radiologic complication rates would be examined; if within normal range, everything would be considered acceptable and focus would be directed elsewhere. If the rate exceeded the standard, the radiologist would bear the consequences. Systems contributions were irrelevant. The doctor was responsible.

In continuous improvement, efforts would be directed toward reducing the existing rate even further, irrespective of the standard, by identifying the wide variety of contributions resulting from the process of providing the radiologic product. The physician's contribution is but a part of the process.

As part of its agenda for change, the Joint Commission for the Accreditation of Healthcare Organizations (JCAHO) is addressing the need to focus on the interrelated processes that impact the delivery of care and on the increased role of top management and medical staff leadership in improving quality rather than just meeting standards. In a critical change, which is consistent with Deming's philosophy, the accreditation manual stresses that quality is an organization-wide responsibility and that most people are motivated and competent in carrying out their assignments. Everyone is responsible for quality and its continuous improvement, not just the QA department or the providers.

JCAHO is formulating new concepts of quality in hospitals that will focus on patient outcomes. How this is achieved is of less importance to the Commission.

Quality Improvement (QI) programs can answer many of the shortcomings of the QA system. QI is developed locally in response to the needs of the organization. It focuses on the process of the delivery of care and in particular acknowledges the need for continual improvement. The system fosters integrated analysis of efficiency and effectiveness. It strives to nurture the professional instinct for continuous self-assessment and improvement among healthcare professionals. It emphasizes supplier–customer relationships and customer satisfaction.

QI recognizes variation over a period of time and encourages evaluation of the pattern of variation, so that appropriate measures toward improvement can be implemented. For example, a film repeat rate of 6% that has been declining over a period of months does not require new corrective measures, whereas a film repeat rate of 6% that has been increasing over several months requires immediate attention.

This all sounds very nice, but how does one go about creating this change in the way business is presently conducted? The transformation to TQM first requires a commitment from top management. Management's adoption of Deming's 14 points provides the method and an appropriate place to start.

DEMING'S 14 POINTS APPLIED TO RADIOLOGY

Any radiology group that has been in practice for long has a plan for where they want to be and how they will reach that goal. Along the way they have adapted to the environment of Medicare/Medicaid, third-party payers, etc. With the latest external influences of diagnosis-related groups and relative value scales, groups that desire to be in business in the next 10 years will likely have to adapt again and readjust their goals.

Some, including the authors, believe that if the continued woes of the healthcare system in the United States are not corrected, a tremendous upheaval in the system will occur, with results that will satisfy no one, unless the leaders in the healthcare industry adopt a plan to redirect that care in a meaningful way. This book is directed toward the implementation of TQM in the practice of radiology as a step in the right direction.

Dr. Deming's 14 points for management (W. Edwards Deming, *Out of the Crisis,* MIT Center for Advanced Engineering Study, Cambridge, Mass., 1986) are discussed here with amplification as they apply to the practice of radiology. The transformation to TQM cannot occur without the leaders of the radiology organization adopting these principles and translating them into action.

In adapting these principles to radiology, the work of Drs. Paul B. Batalden and Loren Vorlicky has been used as a resource and guide.

The 14 Points

1. Create constancy of purpose toward improvement of product and service, with the aim to become competitive and to stay in business and provide jobs.

The radiology practice that wants to be in business in the next 10 to 30 years must be clear today as to why it is in practice and this reason must address the problems it will face staying in practice. Improvement of the service and product each year is essential. If the practice is satisfied with the status quo, there is little likelihood of progress or long-term success. The practice must also have a clear direction for the future in order to adapt to the changes in the healthcare environment and must influence those changes to effect the improvement of medicine through leadership.

Innovation, commitment to research and education, and continuous improvement of the radiologic product lay the foundation upon which the future rests. Constancy of purpose must be communicated to employees, suppliers, and customers. Emphasis on short-term results, which undermine innovation, must be reduced.

2. Adopt a new philosophy.

We are in a new economic age in which the consumer does not have to accept only those products that are available locally. Transportation and competition in imaging have created a marketplace that is driven more and more by the consumer. The consumer can influence who stays in business by choosing a provider. There is likely someone else out there who would very much like to satisfy that patient with their product.

Establishing and meeting standards frequently implies an acceptable rate of defects. Defects, mistakes, improper equipment, and inadequately trained personnel cost money. Radiologists and administrators must take the lead in solving the problems, eliminating the defects, training the people, and continually improving the product.

Running a practice on figures alone undermines the goal of long-term progress. Sometimes doing the right thing, whether or not it fits policy, results in a satisfied customer, from which the "multiplier effect" arises. How many people will the customer tell about his or her great experience?

3. Cease dependence on mass inspection to achieve quality. Build quality into the product in the first place.

Herein lies one of the greatest physician frustrations with QA: The physician innately desires to build quality into his or her product. The rework required by QA is irritating, costly, and does nothing for the patient retrospectively. TQM promotes the idea of allowing the radiologist to build quality into the radiologic product prospectively.

Why are quality control technologists used to ensure that examinations are complete prior to forwarding to the radiologist for interpretation? Instead of someone checking over the work of others, why not train each technologist to quality control his or her own work and put the quality control technologist to work performing examinations or supervising. A side effect of inspection is that it engenders a sense that someone else will find what the originator missed, and therefore less effort and pride are put into the work. A corollary is that if more than one person is responsible, no one is responsible.

If feedback is needed in a system of operation, statistically significant sampling should be conducted, if it is cost effective.

4. End the practice of awarding business on the basis of price alone. Instead, minimize total cost. Move toward a single

supplier for any one item, based on a long-term relationship built on loyalty and trust.

It is likely that each of us at one time or another has purchased something because it was the least expensive, only to have the item fail and require costly repair or replacement. In the life cycle of radiological equipment, it would most likely have been worth buying quality in the first place, even if at a higher initial price, because over the life of the equipment the cost will likely be less than the "low bid." Price has no meaning without quality. Price + Quality = Value.

Communicate your constancy of purpose to suppliers (film, chemistry, equipment, billing, referring physicians, etc.), to the extent possible; choose those that demonstrate statistical control of their product, and develop a long-term relationship with open communication of needs.

Consider this from the perspective of a supplier of healthcare. As Fortune 500 companies apply this principle, will they be looking toward providers that can demonstrate a program of continuous improvement and better quality?

5. Improve constantly and forever the system of production and service, in order to improve quality and productivity and thus constantly reduce costs.

In diagnosis, each patient is unique and therefore each examination is unique. A technologist does not just expose a chest radiograph. The technologist is conducting a test which, if done correctly, will assist the radiologist in rendering a diagnosis for the patient. There is only one chance for optimum success with each patient. This process can be studied and improved.

The process of rendering diagnoses includes many steps taken by referring physicians, patients, techs, and radiologists. There are also many steps in this process which could undergo some improvement. Just ask the referring physician, the patient, the tech, the receptionist, or the radiologist. Or ask the payers. Structure a mechanism to measure and improve these steps—continuously.

Improved total quality means improved productivity and greater market share.

6. Institute training on the job.

In our attention to improving profit, we frequently overlook what makes us profitable—doing things right. If there is too much variation in film density, findings might be missed. If the correct sequence of exams is not followed, the diagnosis may be in doubt or delayed.

Radiologists must have a working knowledge of radiographic positioning and exposure. Technologists must have a working knowledge of the necessity of doing things within a certain uniformity. Reception personnel must have a working knowledge of medical terminology and the preparation requirements of certain exams. All must adopt the constancy of purpose of the organization and the new philosophy of quality improvement.

This requires ongoing education for everyone who participates in the production of the radiologic product, from the receptionist through the billing personnel. The topics must include those which familiarize the employees with:

1. The organization and how their jobs contribute to the constancy of purpose
2. Their responsibilities and the tools to accomplish them
3. Cross training where useful and effective
4. An operational understanding of other job responsibilities
5. Basic statistical control methods

7. *Institute leadership to help people do the job better.*

The philosophy here is that machines are *managed*. People must be *led*. If the radiologist expects to play a leadership role in the radiologic industry, he or she must have the time and be willing to participate in and drive the improvement process. The radiology administrator, as well as the radiologist, must commit his or her time and energy toward assisting workers in accomplishing their responsibilities by:

1. Removing the barriers to pride in accomplishment.
2. Knowing the work they lead people in doing.
3. Recognizing that defects are more likely the fault of the system, and therefore the fault of leadership and management, rather than the willing worker.
4. Listening to the worker when he or she has a suggestion for improvement. The worker is more likely to have better knowledge of the problem.
5. Providing supervisors the time to work with and assist the workers.
6. Appointing supervisors who are well trained in the tasks of their workers, skilled teachers and leaders, and trained in simple statistical methods with the aim of identifying and eliminating special causes of defects and rework.

8. Drive out fear so that everyone can work effectively for the good of the organization.

Fear as a motivator produces short-term results. The long-term losses that an organization suffers from performance impaired by fear outweigh any short-term gains. Continuous improvement by those most likely to know how to improve the process requires the freedom to express and try new ideas. Thought and action must be nourished, not starved. Fear stifles innovation.

Teamwork is essential. The idea that the radiologist is the only person who deserves respect is outmoded. Is the pitcher the most important player on a baseball team? Is the quarterback the most important player on a football team? If the pitcher does not pitch absolutely perfectly, then fielders become important for the success of the team. Similarly, a lone quarterback will find it extremely difficult to win with no receivers or blockers.

The radiology team consists of everyone who participates in the business. Everyone is essential to the continuous improvement of quality and getting the job done. Everyone deserves the respect of others. A caveat to this is that respect is also earned. Each team member has a responsibility to earn respect each day.

9. Break down the barriers between departments.

Create a corporate attitude of service and cooperation toward other departments. Focus improvement efforts on those problems in radiology that affect other departments, but do not expect an immediate return. Assist others in their improvement efforts.

Clinics, wards, nursing staff, admitting, housekeeping, dietary, radiology, pathology, pharmacy, billing, and administration (among others) must interact in order to serve the patient with total quality. All members must be part of the healthcare team. All will find themselves as suppliers and customers in the many cross-functional processes that occur in the course of the daily operation of the facility. Get to know your customer and supplier.

Adversarial relationships are detrimental to the progress of any organization and must be eliminated. Understanding each others' needs and responsibilities is essential.

10. Eliminate slogans, exhortations, and targets for the work force.

Posters and slogans extolling the virtue of zero complaints, worker's pride, etc. are misdirected. Instead of exhorting the receptionists to be polite, the techs to maintain a repeat rate of less than 5%, or the radiologists to sign their reports within 24 hours of the exam, direct your efforts toward the system that most likely created the problem.

Management slogans tend to irritate workers, as do written policies. Every time something goes wrong, another policy is promulgated. Rather than face-to-face interaction to resolve the problem, another policy is issued, which will probably be forgotten or ignored in several weeks. Leadership, on the other hand, would address the constancy of purpose directly to the workers and seek their assistance in resolving issues.

Let the workers create and display their own slogans.

11. Eliminate work quotas. Substitute leadership.

Quotas undermine a sense of quality. Consider an employee who must meet a certain quota each day. This may be reports typed, exam requests entered in a radiology information system, number of chest X-rays performed, number of films interpreted, etc. The quota will usually be met but at the sacrifice of quality. The typist who works at 110 words per minute with 30 errors is probably slower than a typist who works at 55 words per minute with no errors. The time it takes to correct the mistakes is more costly than the slower initial rate.

If a measure of productivity is needed, determine the average output of the product to be measured. Then determine the variation from the average that is acceptable to the organization and the workers. Establish a mechanism to improve the average and reduce the variation by involving the workers responsible for the output. Provide helpful supervision for those who need assistance so that they may improve.

Utilize proven leadership principles in achieving improvements.

12. Eliminate merit rating systems.

Personnel evaluations and merit rating systems undermine pride in workmanship. The efforts of workers too often are directed toward improving their evaluations rather than improving the products for which they are responsible. Rating systems create rivalry, destroy teamwork, build fear, and nurture a sense of short-term accomplishment for quick recognition.

Once again, failure to perform is more often a fault of the system (poor training, inferior machinery, defective materials, etc.), rather than the willing worker. Dr. Deming's 85/15 rule holds that 85% of the problems in an organization are the result of a bad system for which management is responsible. Problems are related to personnel 15% of the time. Grading the person for faults of the system is certainly unfair.

Who wants to be average? Many rating systems require marks such as below average, average, or above average. Who would go to or send their family to an "average" doctor? What professional would admit to being below average? Ridiculous as it seems, if a statistical average can be measured, 50% would be in the lower half. This does not mean that they are bad. Dr. Deming recommends that if a rating system must be used, it should include three categories: (a) does not meet expectations, (b) meets expectations, and (c) exceeds expectations.

13. Institute a vigorous program of education and self-improvement.

A new program of management and leadership in which the participation of all employees is required necessitates education in (1) the new responsibilities brought about by the change, (2) teamwork, and (3) skills maintenance in the wide variety of exams performed in the radiology department. It is recommended that radiologists and radiology administrators take a leadership role in the training of department personnel (both as their customer and as their leader). Training in the basics of statistical techniques is essential.

14. Involve everyone in the organization in the transformation to total quality improvement.

Transformation requires that top management be committed to the change, with a plan of action to involve all people in the organization. Willing workers cannot do it on their own. Radiology administrators cannot do it without the support and commitment of the radiologists. In the hospital, both must have the commitment of the hospital administration.

The preceding 14 points must ultimately be adopted by all in the organization who contribute to its operation.

2

CREATING PURPOSE in the RADIOLOGIC PRACTICE

VISION

Once the upper management of a radiology organization is convinced of the need for a commitment to total quality improvement, implementation of the first of the 14 points is essential. In order to involve everyone in the transformation and make the goals of the organization clear, a well-defined vision and mission must be created. Guiding principles can be used as the foundation upon which the vision and mission are based.

For a perfect example of a vision and mission that create a transformation, we have only to look at the origins of the United States. At a time when the prevailing paradigm of government was a monarchy, learned men of the American colonies used their vision of a desirable and achievable future in identifying "self-evident" truths in the Declaration of Independence. These men transformed the governmental paradigm of rule by divine right to the paradigm of rule by the people.

Organizational vision statements need not be as complex as the documents that founded the United States. In fact, it is preferable that they be simple and easily understood. They should also be energizing. They should provide general standards by which the organization can be measured. They should also define quality and instill the importance of belonging to the organization. These statements should aid in achieving the strategic objectives at all levels of the radiology organization.

It is of utmost importance to the organization that the mission be consistent with the vision and that the guiding principles be consistent with both the vision and the mission. All employees must know and understand the vision, mission, and guiding principles, because it is only through the involvement of everyone that the goals can be realized.

These statements may include the commitment of the organization as well as the expectations of vendors of radiological equipment and supplies. Once again, it is most beneficial to all parties if the visions, missions, and guiding principles of the interacting organizations are consistent and in alignment. One does not need a degree in business administration to recognize that a radiology group with a vision and mission that are counter to the hospital or clinic it serves will not survive. Drafting consistent documents engenders a spirit of cooperation and understanding (Deming point #4).

Guidelines that may be used in drafting a vision statement are as follows:

- Create a statement that describes a possible and desirable future state of being for the practice.
- Allow yourself to visualize new horizons of responsibility for the practice.
- Visualize how you perceive and regard yourself and others in the schema of radiologic practice.
- Visualize how you desire others to perceive and regard your organization.
- Define a target as the ideal you wish to reach.

A vision statement should address the following criteria:

- Embody the constancy of your purpose.
- Be compelling and inspiring, giving meaning and importance to belonging to the practice.
- Be energizing and empowering, creating commitment, enthusiasm, and willingness to work. In creating this atmosphere, the statement must embody values to which those in the practice adhere—personal and professional core values.
- Be easily understood by all members of the department.
- Be simple.
- Be consistent with the vision statement of the parent or major cooperating organization.

Examples

Radiology Department Vision Statement

The Radiology Department strives to provide the highest quality radiologic services as an integral part of the healthcare team while pursuing continuous improvement and innovation.

Amplification: Our goal is to consistently provide the highest quality achievable in the performance of our mission. We wish to be respected and welcome members of the teams of personnel working toward a common goal: successful outcomes in all patient encounters. We plan to achieve this status by continually looking for improvements in our methods and being innovative in our approach to problem solving.

MISSION

From the vision of the U.S. Declaration of Independence, the mission statement was drafted 13 years later in the form of the Constitution. It was and remains the written standard against which all of our laws of governance are measured.

In some business circles, cynical comments may have been made regarding mission and vision statements; however, these comments probably reflect the feelings of individuals dissatisfied with their experience in the organization. This dissatisfaction may arise in an organization that fails to abide by its stated mission. There should be no question that a clear vision, mission, and set of guiding principles, if correctly prepared, will assist in transforming the workplace into a pro-active organization from top to bottom.

Care should be taken in drafting these statements, and input should be obtained from a broad cross section of workers. Guidelines that may be used in preparing a mission statement are as follows:

- Clearly state the intent of the organization.
- Define the product/products.
- Define the scope of individual responsibility.
- Identify the market to which your product is delivered.
- Define the measure of commitment.
- Ensure that the mission is consistent with the vision statement and with the mission of the parent or cooperating organization.

Examples

A very concise statement of purpose which covers the first four attributes of a mission statement is as follows:

We are in business to manufacture and distribute athletic footwear to recreational users.

The following statements are too broad:

Our business is service.
We are in the healthcare business.

The following statements are too narrow:

We distribute jogging shoes.
We provide X-ray reports.

Massachusetts Respiratory Hospital Mission Statement

MRH has been guided by its mission to care for patients with respiratory disease since its founding in 1918. Our focused sense of purpose is a priority for us and is supported by a drive to continuously improve our services.

Radiology Department Mission Statement

We are committed to provide the highest quality service, radiologic diagnosis and therapy, and training in direct support of patient care.

Amplification: Our products are (1) service, (2) diagnosis, (3) treatment, and (4) training. For each we are committed to provide the highest quality to the best of our abilities. We recognize that in the performance of our duties, we must always consider the impact of our service, diagnosis, and treatment decisions on patient care.

GUIDING PRINCIPLES

Immediately upon the adoption of the U.S. Constitution, the framers sensed a need to guarantee certain principles. These guiding principles were provided in the form of the first ten amendments to the Constitution, or the Bill or Rights.

As the Bill of Rights continues to guide us as the core values in our society, guiding principles for an organization provide the strength of timeless values during times of change and help us accept and adapt to change. Security and long-term success are built upon the core principles of any organization. These principles should enhance the flavor of the organization as established by the vision and mission. They further empower employees to carry out the aims of the business without micro-management by providing a frame of reference for each employee to apply to all that is done in the name of the organization.

For example, an unempowered receptionist will have to ask if an intravenous urogram can be scheduled on a weekend. A receptionist empowered by the principle of doing what is in the best interest of the patient will schedule the exam.

Guidelines that may be used in drafting guiding principles are as follows. Guiding principles should

- Identify the core values or principles that will guide you in the performance of your mission
- Define what the organization stands for
- Embody the principles of total quality management
- Be concise (the degree to which they are learned and followed is inversely related to their length)
- Empower people to do their jobs
- Be consistent with the mission and vision of the department and the vision and mission of the organization

Examples

Massachusetts Respiratory Hospital Quality Guidelines

- We are committed to providing the best quality in our services and to designing our services based on customer needs and expectations.
- We seek to continuously improve every process of planning, operations, and service delivery.
- We believe that emphasis on design of improvements, rather than inspection, is a more effective method of achieving quality.
- We seek supervisory and management practices which focus on the improvement of the systems in which people work.
- We believe that people work best in a caring organizational environment that is characterized by trust and integrity.
- We are committed to develop a work environment that relies on cooperation rather than competition.
- We seek an environment where suggestions for improvement and innovation are solicited from patients, employees, and others, where ideas are shared, and where teamwork flourishes.
- We believe that communication by senior management about the goals we seek and information about what progress is being made toward achieving these goals is essential in enlisting effective participation by our employees.

- Recognizing that people are our greatest asset, we wish to create an environment in which our employees are encouraged to seek personal and professional development so that the services they provide will sustain our efforts of continuous improvement.
- We commit to all employees to provide the opportunity to learn about our systems for continuous improvement and to provide opportunities to work together to change the processes with which they work.
- We seek to be a hospital that employees can be proud of and to provide a work environment which encourages all employees to take pride in their work.
- We will endeavor to provide to all employees feedback from customers on the results in order that they may understand and improve our services.
- We want all employees to have a clear understanding of their jobs and their individual roles in improving quality.
- We are committed to the elimination of barriers which have the effect of adding costs through waste, rework, and needless complexity.
- When we can purchase a service or product of better quality, we will never knowingly settle for less.
- We seek suppliers who will be our long-term partners and who will provide us the best service and products at the lowest total cost.
- We create budgets and quantitative estimates of our performance each year to monitor our progress internally and to help us communicate with our external public. We recognize that these targets are not a substitute for methods which help our employees to do their best.
- We seek to become more skillful in our use of statistical thinking and quantitative methods in order to improve what we do.

Radiology Department Guiding Principles

The Radiology Department exists to:

1. Serve the best interests of the patient at all times.
   Amplification: In our daily service efforts we always consider what is in the best interest of the patient.
2. Always care for others in the performance of our duties.
   Amplification: A more pleasant workplace is the result of the mutual respect we show for one another and for those with whom

we interact. We strive to provide understanding and compassion to others in an effort to break down the artificial barriers that exist between departments, sections, divisions, and work centers and to engender a sense of cooperation and teamwork. We must recognize the importance of the customer–supplier relationship in all our interactions and strive at all times to satisfy the customers, giving them what they have the right to expect.

3. Provide for the professional development of all department members.

    Amplification: No job or responsibility in this department is small or insignificant. Everyone is essential in the successful completion of our mission. As such, each individual requires adequate training to provide the tools to accomplish the tasks assigned. As our mission, we are committed to constantly prepare ourselves and others to become self-sufficient in our jobs and assume greater responsibilities. We will provide this through leadership, recognizing that people cannot be forced into perfection, and through education, recognizing that we can only perform our jobs if we are given the tools to succeed.

4. Forever evaluate and improve the processes that define our mission.

    Amplification: We believe that quality is everyone's responsibility and that standards should be set only as a temporary goal; when reached, they should be reset to a point providing greater quality. Only through the careful measurement of our processes can we determine the means of improvement. The quality that we seek is to always exceed and improve upon current applicable standards. In this improvement process, we must recognize the importance of the customer–supplier relationship and improve these interactions.

5. Integrate service, training, and research to achieve the best outcome for all who seek our assistance.

    Amplification: In spite of the remarkable advances in diagnostic technologies in recent decades, much about the practice of medicine remains unknown. As professionals, it is our legacy to those who will follow in our footsteps to gather the information we can obtain from our daily practices and apply this information in the improvement process. More often than not, healthcare encounters are finite periods, defined by a beginning at presentation and progressing to an end at treatment, at which time the result or outcome can be measured. What has not been examined well in the past is what people and resources were used in the process of moving from presentation to the end of treatment. Studying this process can provide us a measure of how the practice of medicine may be optimized. We accept this study as part of our mission and as essential to the survival of the profession as we know it.

3

SEEKING
CONTINUOUS IMPROVEMENT

WHAT THE CUSTOMER WANTS

*...defects and faults that get into the hands of the customers lose
the market and cost him his job.*

W. Edwards Deming

How the customer fits into the total quality concept is discussed in this
chapter. Bear in mind that this "customer" is not necessarily the traditional end user of the product. There are internal and external customers
who need satisfaction, as well as the "ultimate" consumer of the product
or service. In radiology there may well be multiple simultaneous customers (patient, referring physician, payers, even others within the radiology
department).

A simplistic way of stating the premise of this chapter is (1) identify
the customer, (2) determine the customer needs and wants, and (3)
provide them and forever improve upon them. This is the mechanism
that leads to reduced waste and unreimbursable expenses and increased
profits, as well as attracting new business by providing high quality.

Quality has many facets but can be defined as meeting or exceeding
the needs and expectations of the customer, delighting the customer,
and providing what he or she wants or needs. Identification of the
customer is the first step in the quality improvement process. The
customer of a radiology service may be a person, a department, or an
organization. This includes patients and their families, physicians, hospitals, hospital employees, departments, department employees, and
payers. Satisfaction of these "customers" may be as sophisticated as the
rapid and accurate diagnosis of an affliction or as simple as the

25

radiologist's participation in housekeeping's hazardous waste program by disposing of used syringes and soiled sponges in hazardous waste receptacles. In each example there is a customer to satisfy. The breadth of these examples demonstrates the commitment to *total* quality.

Understanding the customer's opinion regarding quality of services is an essential part of quality improvement. Various levels of customer expectations can be broadly classified:

- **Level 1:** The service meets the basic assumed level of quality. *Examples:* The physician expects to receive a radiology report within 24 hours. The patient assumes that the correct radiology examination will be performed.
- **Level 2:** This is an intermediate level of satisfaction for the customer. *Examples:* The physician expects a written report within 24 hours but receives a telephone call immediately after the radiological exam to inform him or her of unexpected findings. The patient received prompt attention at the reception desk and the radiology examination was carried out in a timely fashion.
- **Level 3:** The customer's highest level of expectation is met. *Examples:* The patient was satisfied with prompt, courteous attention by the radiology reception staff, was delighted with the caring and courteous treatment during the examination, and was pleased with receiving the health education pamphlet regarding the exam.

Because the customer's needs and expectations are always changing, capturing this information is a dynamic process. An appropriate questionnaire may be used to obtain accurate and reliable data on customer needs and expectations and judgment of the quality of service provided. Because the radiology service has many different customers, different sets of questions must be designed for different groups.

For a questionnaire to produce valid and reliable information and have a high response rate, the information gathering form should have the following characteristics:

1. It should be self-administered.
2. It should be short, precise, and concise and ideally should require less than 15 minutes to complete.
3. The same set of questions should be asked of all respondents.
4. Each question should be clearly stated and carry the same meaning for every respondent.
5. It should include background variables.
6. Questions must be quantitative, allowing for multiple choices.

Wording of questions is obviously very important. Good questions should:

1. Maximize the relationship between the answers and what the researcher is trying to measure.
2. Lead to consistent answers in comparable situations.
3. Have a predictable relationship to facts or subjective states that are of interest.
4. Minimize a sense of judgment.

While quality in the healthcare setting is difficult to define, the data collected over time from a well-constructed questionnaire provide a valuable measure of quality.

Example 1

How would you describe the waiting time before your radiology examination?

(1) Very long   (2) Moderately long   (3) Satisfactory

This question is vague. Responses would be very difficult to analyze, and standard responses are unlikely. A better question would be

The waiting time between your arrival at the radiology department and the start of your examination was:

(1) 1–10 minutes   (3) 21–30 minutes
(2) 11–20 minutes   (4) More than 30 minutes

Example 2

How would you grade the quality of service provided by the radiology staff on a scale of 1 to 10, 1 being poor and 10 being excellent.

This question is ambiguous. Are clerical or technical staff or the radiologist's service being graded? The background, biases, and educational level of the respondent will influence the answer. Responses will be difficult to analyze. A better question would be

How would you rate the following qualities of the radiology technologist? (Please circle the appropriate answer: 1= very good, 2 = good, 3 = poor.)

(a) Caring	1	2	3
(b) Courtesy	1	2	3
(c) Professional appearance	1	2	3

Trends in customer rating of quality should lead to identification of those services where the opportunity for improvement exists. Assessment of customer needs provides direction for future planning.

Providing for the customer's needs and wants is the subject of this chapter. The discussion will be restricted to examples of measuring quality. These measurements are divided into departmental logistics (focusing on acquiring the examination, providing service, and distributing the product) and the clinical science of diagnosis.

Understanding measurement is critical to defining and improving quality. Terms encountered in the measurement of quality are quality characteristics, key quality characteristics, process variables, and key process variables.

Characteristics of the radiology service that are important to the customer constitute *quality characteristics*. This is how the customer would identify his or her needs and expectations regarding radiology service. *Key Quality Characteristics* (KQCs) are those quality characteristics that are most important to the customer.

Recognizing that some variation is normal, *process variables* are those factors that create variation in the every-day performance of operations. Manpower, machines, materials, methods, environment, and measurements all contribute to variation. *Key Process Variables* (KPVs) are those components of a process that have a cause-and-effect relationship with the KQCs, such that manipulation and control of the KPV will change the variation of the KQC and/or change its average value.

Methods for defining and measuring quality as well as identifying KQCs and KPVs will be discussed in Chapter 4, along with a description of the basic process. What follows here is an amplification of what can be measured in the radiology department to identify areas for improvement.

MEASURABLE DEPARTMENT LOGISTICS

A myriad of processes in the radiology department can cause any number of "problems" that affect customer satisfaction. Some of the logistic characteristics of the department that can help define the quality of the customer's experience are reviewed in this section. The participation of the radiologist in these types of issues is essential if leadership in the profession is to be maintained.

When measuring quality characteristics of the department, the sample size must be considered. Measuring every item may be time and cost prohibitive. Too few samples will be meaningless. Those intrepid souls

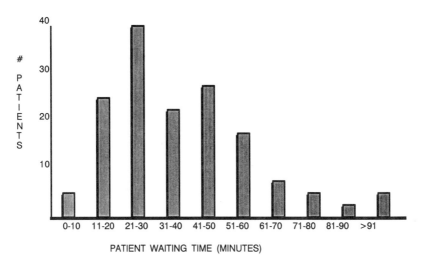

Figure 3.1 Histogram of Patient Waiting Times

who desire more information on meaningful sampling are referred to Chapter 6.

In the examples that follow, no conclusion should be drawn as to the satisfactory or unsatisfactory nature of the values. The customer determines what is satisfactory or unsatisfactory. The purpose is continuous improvement, as opposed to meeting some random standard.

Patient Waiting Time

One of the most frequently encountered problems is the excessive length of time the patient waits in the department for an exam. Obviously, recording the time the patient arrives and the time the patient leaves will measure the waiting time (see Figure 3.1). However, a more detailed analysis is necessary in order to improve waiting time.

Patient waiting time will be used as a sample quality characteristic throughout Chapters 3–6 to illustrate the concepts and tools of total quality management.

The frequency distribution of waiting times is demonstrated in Figure 3.1. It indicates that the most frequent wait was from 11 to 20 minutes. The average of this frequency distribution, however, is about 42 minutes. This is certainly a measure that customers will appreciate. In order to improve this value, more detailed information is needed to indicate where the slowest portions of the imaging sequence are located. This process is called *stratification*. How the measurements are broken down

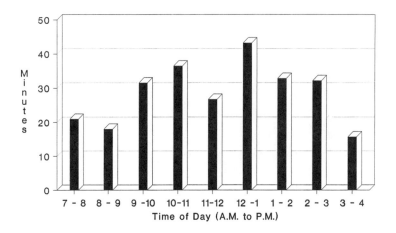

Figure 3.2 Time from Reception to Entering Exam Room by Time of Day

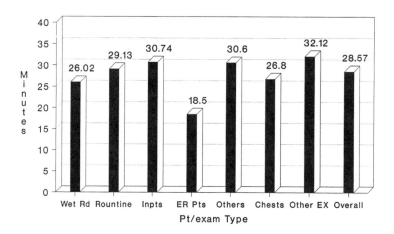

Figure 3.3 Time from Reception to Entering Exam Room by Patient/Exam Type

will be determined by the flow of the operation. Figures 3.2 and 3.3 illustrate sample times from patient check-in until entering the exam room. In general, this shows an increase through the middle part of the day, when patient load is greatest. The data are further divided by patient and exam types as well as time of day.

Check-in waiting time versus patient type or exam type is shown in Figure 3.3. This illustrates that emergency room patients receive faster service than others in the reception process.

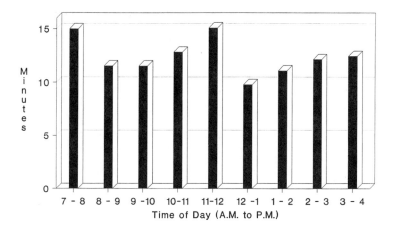

Figure 3.4 Time from Patient Entering X-ray Room to Exam Completed by Time of Day

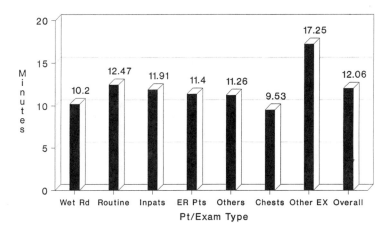

Figure 3.5 Time from Entering X-ray Room to Exam Completely Processed by Patient Type/Patient Exam

The time it takes to position the patient, expose the films, process them, and check them for quality is shown in Figures 3.4 and 3.5. There is little variation for time of day or patient/exam type, which is expected. Chest radiographs take less time, as reflected here.

Figures 3.6 and 3.7 show the composite time it takes to match the exam with the film jacket, to reach the radiologist, and for the radiologist to read the film and write a brief report. In this example, it takes almost an hour for the exam to be read, so the patient could leave with a report after the noon hour. The delay in obtaining the reading is most likely

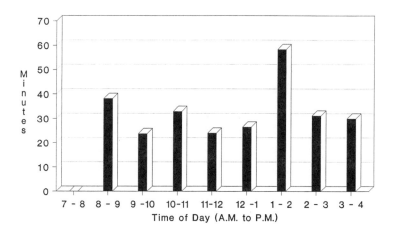

Figure 3.6 Time from Patient Entering X-ray Room to Exam Completed by Time of Day (no sampling for 7–8)

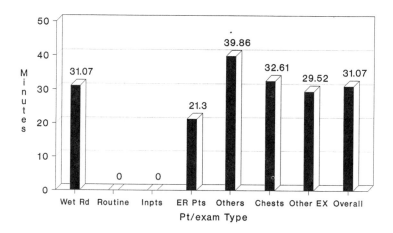

Figure 3.7 Routines and Inpatients Examined Separately (reading time once exam complete includes time to match old film)

the result of a special cause which, when investigated, can be easily corrected. An example of a special cause may be that the radiologist left the department for lunch. The problem of obtaining readings during the lunch hour can be corrected by making a different arrangement for readings during this time.

Referring to Figure 3.7, it can also be seen from the data that emergency room patients receive appropriate attention in that their readings take less time than those of other patient types.

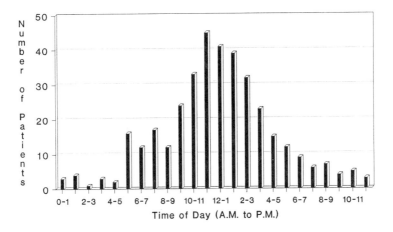

Figure 3.8 Time from Reception to Entering Exam Room by Time of Day

The breakdown of the data can easily be performed by a personal computer using a database. Sorting the database by different factors (such as time of day, patient type, exam type, day of the week, etc.) will provide good information that can be used to seek improvement by focusing on the factor that most significantly contributes to less than optimal quality. In this example, attention may be directed toward decreasing the reception and reading time by studying each process in further detail. Other examples of quality characteristics and process variables that can be measured are as follows:

"Walk-in" Patient Workload by Hour

Knowing the number of people who present each hour for exams will help in managing the service. This seems like common sense, but having the appropriate data will be important in acquiring the necessary personnel or supporting innovative changes in work schedules to accommodate people who need to be examined before or after work. For example, as shown in Figure 3.8, a workload peak in the middle of the day may require supervisors to perform examinations during the peak work load or necessitate hiring of part-time technologists to work during those periods.

Exam Time for Radiologic Procedures

The patient throughput will determine the maximum number of patients that can be imaged in a given time period. Studying the exam process can reduce the amount of time spent completing the exam, which will improve patient throughput.

Fluoroscopy Time per Exam

In keeping with the good radiologic practice of maintaining the exposure as low as reasonably achievable (ALARA), finding ways to reduce the average fluoroscopy time per exam will improve quality and will reduce use of the anodes.

Backlog of Scheduled Exams

Knowing how long it will take before a patient can schedule an exam will support opening additional shifts or obtaining additional imaging capacity.

Report Availability Time

Satisfying the patient accomplishes nothing for the referring physician if a report is not quickly made available. There must be no delay when therapeutic decisions are awaiting the radiologist's assessment.

Acquisition of Patient Information for Exams Requested

This is inordinately helpful to the radiologist and the patient because often the exam can be tailored to the information required. This *a priori* information very often improves confidence in the diagnosis.

Film Waste Rate

This can always be improved. An increase in the rate is usually due to a special cause.

Exam Repeat Rate

This also can always be improved. Rework is expensive.

Cost per Exam

There is a great deal of waste in radiologic practice. Prepackaged trays sometimes contain more items than are needed and the excess ends up being discarded. By decreasing cost, the department or practice can remain competitive.

Radiographic Exams Ordered but Not Performed

This is a major problem in terms of credibility and reliability.

Radiographic Exams Completed but Not Interpreted

This is a drain on profitability.

Number of Exams Performed by Type and Requesting Location

This is a great tool for utilization and marketing.

Safety Violations or Hazards Encountered

Correcting hazards is everyone's responsibility. A program to identify and study hazardous conditions in order to minimize their impact on patients and workers is essential. If management does not care, why should the workers? If the leadership cares, so will the workers.

A good example was provided by Dr. David Garvin (our boss), Director of Ancillary Services at the National Naval Medical Center. Paper clips have a way of decreasing the life cycle of vacuum cleaners, so housekeeping requested that everyone try to keep them off the floors. While walking through the department one day, we walked by a wad of paper and a paper clip errantly placed near the wall. Dr. Garvin stooped, picked it up, and dropped it into the nearest receptacle. What we took away from this is that leadership must set the example in order to expect others to do what is requested.

Patient Complaints/Compliments and Surveys

Every complaint should be investigated and resolved. Trending is needed. Compliments should be publicly passed on to those responsible. Discipline and redirection should be discussed behind closed doors.

Number of Phone Calls through Reception

Busy people do not like to spend a long time listening to the phone ring on the other end, because this is wasted time. The unanswered phone engenders a perception of poor professionalism of the party being called. Are more phone lines needed? Are unnecessary calls that could be redirected clogging the lines? As an example, call several highly successful companies and count the number of rings before the phone is answered. Then call several failing companies and count the number of rings.

Number of Incomplete/Illegible Requests

This is admittedly a supplier issue. If it is a problem, it must be addressed. Incorrect exams, wrong patients, and inaccurate diagnoses can result.

Others

Other quality characteristics that can be measured include:

- CPT coding accuracy
- Stock shortages and overstocking
- Computer down time
- Expired materials
- Amount of overtime
- Room inventories
- "Crash cart" inventories
- Film check-out frequency
- Film jacket filing time
- Film jacket retrieval time
- Film check-out delinquency rate

MEASURABLE RADIOLOGIC SCIENCE

A review of the science of diagnostic imaging in disease populations is provided in this section. Statistical factors that influence the diagnostic capability of exams will be reviewed, showing how these factors influence medical decision making.

In today's highly competitive medical marketplace it is not enough to "lay eyes" on film and produce a report in order to be a diagnostic radiologist. It is our responsibility to provide diagnostic service to our referring physicians and in doing so assist them in making the decisions necessary for a successful outcome in a disease process. Yet, as always, our ultimate service is to the patient.

Disease Populations

The intent of diagnostic radiology is to find some discriminating factor or group of factors in a radiologic examination that can be used to determine the presence or absence of disease. The good news is that fairly reliable discriminating factors exist to detect disease. The bad news is that they are not perfect.

If a population histogram of patients with and without disease were displayed, with the horizontal axis as the discriminating factor (e.g., cardiothoracic ratio relating to heart disease) as in Figure 3.9, instead of these population sets being distinct, they would overlap to some extent. Thus, normal patients fall into the disease measurement range and abnormal patients fall into the non-disease range. This is a fact of life in the laboratory as well as diagnostic radiology. There are very few perfect diagnostic discriminators.

Diagnostic Assessment

Diagnostic examinations must undergo rigorous testing to determine their ability to detect abnormality. In the spirit of continuous improvement, diagnosticians should also undergo continual self-assessment to improve their ability to detect abnormality. Each can be evaluated by a simple results table (Figure 3.10).

Any objective measurement of diagnostic performance must evaluate the agreement between the diagnosis rendered by the imaging system and some external standard of truth. The vertical axis is the truth axis here. The presence or absence of disease must be determined using some "gold standard" that is assumed to be perfectly truthful. This is usually tissue proof of disease or long-term outcome suggesting the absence of disease.

The horizontal axis is the test (exam) result (positive or negative). The results are a function of the following:

1. The exam being properly conducted
2. Defining the radiographic presentation of disease
3. Setting the appropriate threshold for positive/negative
4. The eye detecting the radiographic presentation
5. Proper interpretation of the finding

Where there is agreement between the truth axis and the test axis, "true" positives (TP) and "true" negatives (TN) exist. When there is disagreement, "false" positives (FP) and "false" negatives (FN) exist. Another category should be added to any evaluation of a diagnostic test: *indeterminate*. This is used for exams that do not determine positive or negative. This category is frequently missing from the professional literature but is essential in the evaluation of exam utility. An exam that has a high percentage of indeterminate results would be a poor screening tool and of little value to the patient and referring physicians.

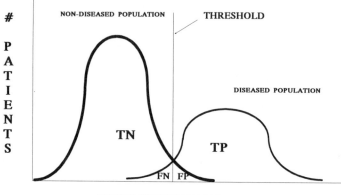

Figure 3.9 Overlapping Population Sets

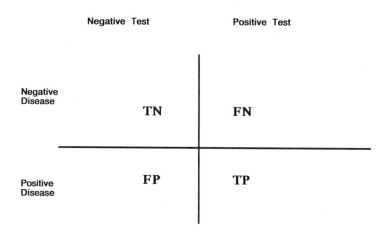

Figure 3.10 Results Table

Definitions of Exam Capability

Sensitivity: TP/(TP + FN). The ability to detect an abnormality by exam, given that it is present in the patient.

Specificity: TN/(TN + FP). The ability to determine normal by exam when the patient is truly free of disease or to differentiate one disease from another.

Accuracy: (TP + TN)/(TP + TN + FP + FN). The percentage of correct tests.

Positive Predictive Value: TP/(TP + FP). The likelihood that the patient has the disease in question, given that there is a positive test result.

Negative Predictive Value: TN/(TN + FN). The likelihood that the patient is free of the disease in question, given that there is a negative test result.

Exam (Test) Value

Sensitivity and *specificity* are measures of the effectiveness of the exam in identifying abnormality and normality, respectively. They are of great value in comparing one diagnostic test to another but of little value to the referring physician in therapeutic decision making. However, knowledge of these values is useful in selecting the most helpful exam to evaluate the presence or absence of disease.

Accuracy is of little scientific merit when applied to population sets. Very high or very low disease rates will naturally have high accuracy regardless of the effectiveness of the exam.

Of more value to the clinician in therapeutic decision making are the *positive* and *negative predictive values*. These values state the likelihood that a positive or negative exam indicates the presence or absence, respectively, of disease. This is in contradistinction to sensitivity and specificity, which indicate the likelihood that a diseased or non-diseased patient will have a positive or negative exam. This is a subtle but very meaningful difference. Knowledge of predictive values will assist in medical decision making (whether sufficient diagnostic certainty exists to begin treatment of the patient or whether continued testing will improve the diagnostic certainty prior to treatment).

Another way of communicating the validity of examinations to referring physicians is to compute the False-Positive Rate (FPR) and False-Negative Rate (FNR). These are the probabilistic alter egos of the Positive Predictive Value (PPV) and the Negative Predictive Value (NPV).

$$FPR = 1 - PPV \quad FNR = 1 - NPV$$

Note: FPR and FNR are sometimes defined as (1 − specificity) and (1 − sensitivity), respectively. These are pre-test ratios and should not be confused with the terms used above, which are the result of the outcome of the test (post-test).

Exam Value as a Function of Threshold

Threshold is defined as the point along a continuum of values at either side of which a diagnostician determines that there is a significant likelihood of the presence or absence of disease.

Changing the threshold for a positive test in order to improve detection of disease will result in greater sensitivity, but will usually increase the number of false positives as well. The associated specificity may fall. An example of when this would be helpful is in a clinical setting where the lack of treatment is devastating, but there is less harm in treating a false positive (e.g., infantile pneumonia, scurvy, ectopic pregnancy).

Moving the threshold to allow for fewer positive exams will decrease the sensitivity, decrease the number of false positives, and improve specificity. This situation is warranted in cases where the treatment can be devastating and the number of false positives should be minimized (e.g., brain stem lesions and bone tumors).

Exam Value as a Function of Prevalence

Both predictive values and post-test false rates are functions of the prevalence of disease as well as the sensitivity and specificity of the examination. For example, in a setting of low disease prevalence such as a screening examination, the positive predictive value of the exam would be very low and the false-positive rate would be increased.

In a setting where the prevalence is high (e.g., patients preselected for the exam by the use of clinical indicators), the positive predictive value is greater (but still somewhat dependent on the sensitivity of the exam) and the false-positive rate declines. Conversely, the negative predictive value is very high when disease prevalence is low and is lower when disease prevalence is high.

This does not, however, get us off the hook when playing the game of absolutes with a patient. Many patients with disease expect that a diagnostic exam will detect the abnormality and that the absence of abnormality means a "clean bill of health." Care must be taken so as not to perpetuate this myth.

Continuous quality improvement can be applied to radiologic science to achieve the following benefits:

1. Improve sensitivity and specificity of the diagnostic system (this implies that the radiologist and the diagnostic machine are one radiologic unit).
2. Find additional radiologic signs to improve the sensitivity and specificity of examinations.

3. Evaluate clinical indicators that improve the diagnostic yield or obviate the need for high-volume or high-cost exams.
4. Evaluate the impact or contribution of specific exams on patient outcomes.
5. Determine the utility of moving disease detectability thresholds for better patient outcomes.
6. Improve complication rates for invasive or intrusive procedures.
7. Improve positive biopsy rates.
8. Maximize the utility of radiologic equipment while maintaining detectability of disease (e.g., can 10-mm CT or MR slices determine the same information as 5-mm or 1.5-mm cuts).
9. Use of non-invasive procedures to improve patient outcomes.
10. Improve radiologic diagnosis with pathologic correlation.
11. Minimize inter-observer variability, which is common between radiologists.

Many of these issues above can be considered key quality characteristics of the clinical radiologic practice.

SUMMARY

Customers, both internal and external, were identified as the drivers of continuous improvement. The characteristics that may satisfy customers and how to obtain this information was reviewed. How the practice can define its mechanisms or processes for delivery of care so as to further define quality will be presented in Chapter 4. A structured process for problem identification and solution will then be introduced.

4

DEFINING PROCESS
and the TQM METHOD

Every activity, every job is a part of a process.

W. Edwards Deming

The process is the source of an overwhelming number of problems found in business today. Less successful businesses lack knowledge about how their processes operate and lack the insight necessary to improve their processes by knowing how they should work. Errors occur in carrying out the established procedures, unnecessary steps waste resources, variations in inputs and outputs increase the tolerances of what is defined as quality, and a lack of preventive measures is built into the steps required to produce the output. The process will be defined in this chapter, and ways to overcome these problems will be introduced.

THE BASIC PROCESS

A process is defined as a series of actions which repeatedly come together to transform inputs into outputs. Processes can be simple or complex, consisting of a series of simple processes. The simple process consists of:

1. Supplier
2. Input
3. Action
4. Output
5. Customer

Virtually any activity can be defined in this way, and one person (the "owner") can be identified as having responsibility and authority for the continuing improvement of that process.

For example, requests for radiographic exams can be defined as follows:

1. Supplier: Referring physician's office
2. Input: Patient information and exam requested
3. Action: Prepare legible request
4. Output: Completed request for exam
5. Customer: Radiology receptionist, patient

Subsequent to this simple process, the larger process of producing the exam and a diagnostic report continues. The receptionist becomes a supplier, providing documentation to the technologist as a customer, who in turn supplies a quality examination to the radiologist as a customer, and so forth, until the patient and referring physician are served as customers.

As this scenario demonstrates, activities in a radiology department are interrelated processes, where the customer of one process is often the supplier of inputs to another process. Actions frequently have more than one customer, and inputs can be received from multiple suppliers. In addition, this example illustrates the concept of "internal" and "external" customers. Serving the patient in the department is likely to be a parallel process.

In further defining the basic process, it is important to recognize (1) the characteristics of the output that satisfy the customer and (2) the factors of the input and action that create variability which influences the output.

Output Quality Characteristics

The basic process can be depicted as follows:

Supplier
Input
Action

Output (characteristics that satisfy the customer)
Customer

Recall from Chapter 3 that quality is primarily determined by the customer and by the innovative thinking of those familiar with the customer's needs. Characteristics of quality can be identified for each process for which there is an identifiable customer, whether internal or external. Once these are established, the Key Quality Characteristics (KQCs) with the strongest influence on customer satisfaction can be selected for measurement and analysis.

Four Steps to Define and Measure Quality

Step 1: Define a process (supplier, input, action, output, customer).

Step 2: Identify a KQC (what is most important to the customer). This requires information about the customer's needs and expectations. This information may be obtained by collecting data with a questionnaire or by measuring the patient's value of the quality characteristic.

Step 3: Define the KQC in terms of how it can be measured (an operational definition). Implementing this step requires thorough knowledge of the services provided by the radiology department as they relate to the KQC and clearly defining how to measure the KQC.

Step 4: Create a data collection plan and implement it. Knowledge of data collection is the key to this step.

Deming (*Out of the Crisis,* MIT Center for Advanced Engineering Study, Cambridge, Mass., 1986) describes an operational definition as "one that people can do business with. An operational definition of safe, round reliable, or any other quality must be communicable, with the same meaning to the vendor as to the purchaser, same meaning yesterday and today to the production worker. Example:

1. A specific test of a piece of material or an assembly
2. A criterion (or criteria) for judgment
3. Decision: yes or no, the object or the material did or did not meet the criterion (or criteria)...."

The data collected for each KQC allow evaluation of how the particular service meets the customer's expectations. Evaluation of data will also reveal the level of customer expectation being met by the service. In keeping with our example of patient waiting time as the global quality characteristic (as discussed in Chapter 3), the overall average waiting time was greater than 40 minutes. Measuring patient waiting time as the difference between the time the patient arrives and leaves reveals little about how to improve this value. More detailed information is needed, such as a breakdown of the times at certain stops along the process of obtaining an X-ray and reading it.

This information is derived by operationally defining the processes that occurred in getting the patient into the room and identifying suppliers, inputs, actions taken by the suppliers, outputs, and the customers of the outputs:

1. Supplier: Receptionists
2. Input: Patient/exam info
3. Action: Computer entry and form completion
4. Output: Completed paperwork
5. Customer: Floor supervisor, patient

The KQCs include (1) accurately completed paperwork and (2) minimum processing time. The time will be considered as the KQC here. Measuring patient waiting time as the difference between the time the patient arrives and leaves reveals nothing about the lag in time from reception desk to exam room. Therefore, this measurement must be stratified into time from check-in to exam room, as in the previous example. Processing time from check-in to arrival in the exam room is from 20 to 40 minutes, with an average of 30 minutes.

Astute managers will note that the first basic process extends to the floor supervisor who assigns the exam to a room. It does not go so far as to get the patient into the room. Therefore:

1. Supplier: Floor supervisor
2. Input: Knowledge of priorities, rooms, work load, and exam needs
3. Action: Room assignments, patient instruction
4. Output: Patient assigned a room ready for exam
5. Customer: Patient, technologist

The KQCs here might be (1) keeping rooms filled with patients and (2) the time elapsed in making assignments. The time from reception to assignment is the measurement made. Further stratification may be necessary to improve this (i.e., measuring the reception processing time and the room assignment time separately).

Process Variables

The basic process can be depicted as follows:

Supplier	(variable factors
Input	influencing
Action	the output)
———	
Output	
Customer	

Factors that have an impact on quality include manpower, machines, materials, methods or procedures, environment, and policies. Those factors of variability that occur within the process can be identified as sources for change in the supplier, input, action portion of the process which may improve the quality characteristics of the output. From these variables, Key Process Variables (KPVs) that will most influence the KQCs can be selected.

Common (random) variation is inherent in the process and cannot be controlled by changing steps in the process. These are variables that occur naturally and over which we have little control. However, *special variation* is a change in definition of the process and the methods of completing the steps, and we do have some measure of control here. These variations can be caused by inadequate training of workers, some unusual occurrence, or special circumstances.

Misidentifying random variation as a special cause leads to tampering with a system that does not need help. Tampering increases variation and results in loss of control. Misidentifying a special cause as a random variation results in undercontrolling a system that needs intervention to regain control.

If the causes of variation in a process are constant, then measuring the outcome will produce a set of data points that have a predictable center (average), central tendency (mode), spread (standard deviation), and shape (skew) that can be mathematically modeled. Data points that fall outside of this model are most likely due to a special cause that requires intervention (i.e., training, increased supervision, identification of a previously unknown cause). These examples all support the theory that identification of problems carries the information needed to solve them.

Note: Increased supervision is not necessarily bad. There is variation in the workplace in terms of the skills and capabilities of all workers. If an average worker can be defined, some will be above average, some average, and some below average, but all contribute to the mission of the organization. Physicians and administrators need to expunge the negative connotation of "below average." In science and statistics, below average carries no subjective judgment. The supervisor's responsibility should be to assist the worker who does not meet expectations.

Five Steps to Identify and Measure Process Variables

Step 1: Brainstorm with workers to identify factors that produce variability in the selected KQC. This is also an operational definition. Try to categorize them as to manpower, machines, materials, methods or procedures, environment, and policies. Apply each to a cause-and-effect diagram.

Step 2: Choose the process variables (KPVs) you theorize will have the greatest impact on the KQC. Choose one KPV that will have the greatest impact. The workers will likely know the right one. If there is disagreement, you may need to use the Pareto chart (see Figure 4.6) to help determine the most important one.

Step 3: Define the KPVs in terms of how they can be measured. Implementation of this step requires thorough knowledge of the services provided by the radiology department as they relate to the KQC and KPV.

Step 4: Devise a plan to measure the KQC and KPV simultaneously, and test your theory of the relationship between them.

Step 5: Plot the results on a scatter diagram (see Figure 4.7).

The activities to be improved can be defined by using these five steps and the KQCs and KPVs can be measured, providing the statistical benchmark needed to begin the improvement process.

In the previous example of patient waiting time, variables such as inoperative equipment, inadequate number of cassettes, slow processors, insufficient number of technologists, moving emergency room patients ahead of routines, and front desk interruptions all contributed to increased waiting time in theory (Figure 4.1). Let's assume that we want to measure the number of technologists (KPV) versus time in check-in room (KQC) to determine if room assignment was delayed by patients waiting for techs to become available.

By measuring waiting times during specified periods with differing numbers of techs available and then correcting for the presented work load, we can determine if there is any relationship between the two. A negative relationship is demonstrated in Figure 4.2. As expected if tech staffing is the problem, patient check-in room waiting time declined with an increased number of techs.

Undertaking quality improvement in this way will produce improved results if a structured plan for problem solving is carried out. Drs. Paul Batalden and Tom Gillem of the Hospital Corporation of America have adapted the quality improvement cycle first espoused by Dr. Shewhart for planning the change for improvement, making the change, observing the effects of the change, and acting to hold the gains or redirect the efforts of improvement (Plan, Do, Check, Act). They prefaced this by FOCUS:

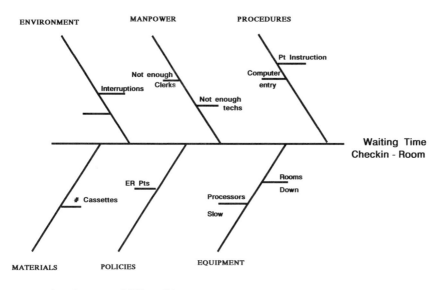

Figure 4.1 Cause-and-Effect Diagram

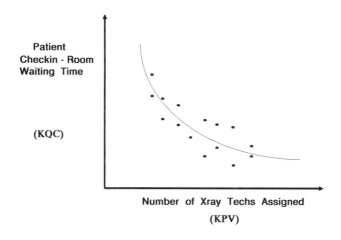

Figure 4.2 Scatter Diagram

Find a problem to solve or a process to improve
Organize a team that knows the process
Clarify current knowledge of the process
Understand causes of process variation
Select the process improvement

Plan the implementation and continue data collection
Do the improvements
Check the results
Act to hold the gains and continue improvement

FOCUS-PDCA is a structured problem-solving process that provides a road map for continuous improvement. It will be discussed in detail throughout the following section.

This may seem compulsive to many. It is, but the results cannot be denied. Many in American industry who have tried to shortcut the process in order to obtain instant results end up with long-term setbacks. The Americans and Japanese who derived these methods took over 30 years to arrive at them. We have the benefit of learning from them in a small fraction of the time. Implementing change takes courage and persistence.

FOCUS-PDCA

F (Find a Problem to Improve and Define It)

The following considerations are helpful in selecting a quality improvement project in the early stages of implementing TQM:

1. Improving the project should result in improved operations.
2. Improving the project should be achievable and should have a good chance of success.
3. The process to be improved should be repeated in a fairly fast cycle (should produce more than a few data points per month).
4. The size of the project should not be too large so as to be unmanageable or so small that no one will notice if improvements are made.
5. The project should address something that is important to the customer.
6. The owner of the process should always be a member of the team.

Follow-up projects can examine longer term issues such as return on investment, defining what "future state-of-the-art" imaging will mean for patients and their long-term outcomes, interdisciplinary activities that improve outcomes, and innovative solutions to difficult diagnostic problems. For a more detailed discussion of these issues, see Chapter 7.

The Pareto (pa-ray-toe) chart (see Figure 4.6) is particularly helpful in determining the most significant problems to tackle. It diagrammatically represents the most pressing problems.

Once a problem is identified, it should be defined by a statement of opportunity which:

1. Describes the mission or intent of the improvement effort
2. Defines the symptoms of the problem in specific and measurable terms
3. Describes the problem in terms of performance (what is the current impact and who or what will benefit)
4. Defines the boundaries of the problem being studied
5. Does not include preconceived root causes or implied solutions and does not affix blame
6. Describes why it is important that this problem be solved now

Tools commonly employed in identifying and defining problems (further explanation of these tools can be found in Chapter 5) include:

- Brainstorming
- Data collection
- Pareto chart (see Figure 4.6)
- Flowchart (see Figure 4.3)

O (Organize a Team to Work on Improvement)

Who best knows the process identified in **F** (find a problem) and who interacts in the process of achieving the output? This includes supplier–customer relationships throughout the process. A *team leader* should be selected from this group. This person retains most of the "ownership" of the process and is responsible for providing direction, initiating activities, encouraging members, and leading meetings.

The leader may want other members of the team to assume roles, including a timekeeper, a recorder, and a facilitator/advisor who helps members stay true to the process of seeking quality improvement. (For further discussion on leading team meetings, refer to Peter R. Scholtes, *The Team Handbook: How to Improve Quality with Teams,* Joiner Associates, Madison, Wisc., 1988.)

Tools commonly employed in teams within an organization include:

- Brainstorming
- Flowchart (see Figure 4.3)

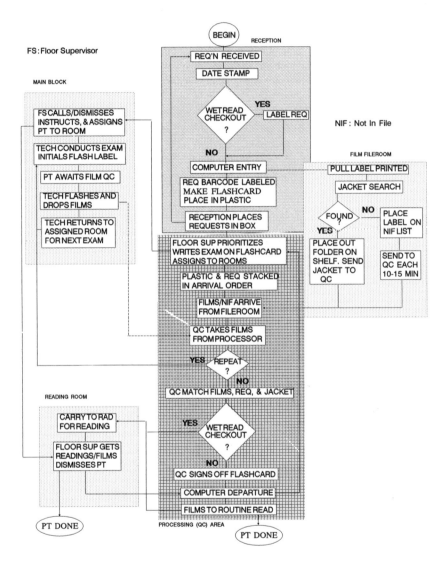

Figure 4.3 Patient Throughput Flowchart

C (Clarify the Problem and Current Knowledge of the Process)

Identify the entire process within the boundary conditions set by the opportunity statement. Chart the process as it currently operates from start to finish. A sample flowchart for a radiology department is provided in Figure 4.3. (For a more detailed discussion of flowcharts, see Chapter 5.) The process being charted is likely to be a series of the basic processes defined earlier in this chapter (supplier, input, action, output, customer), as illustrated in Figure 4.4.

Identify the needs and expectations of each "customer" of each basic process identified in the overall flowchart, and then determine which of these needs and expectations (quality characteristics) most strongly influence improvement. These needs and expectations are the KQCs.

Once agreement on the definition of the process is reached, verify that the opportunity statement and the team are applicable. Are there any obvious improvements that can be made? Are data needed to further define the process? If there is variation from one person to another as to how the process works, how does this impact the operation? Is refinement needed? If progress is stalled, the opportunity statement, the team membership, and the process defined here may be out of alignment.

Tools commonly employed in process clarification include:

- Data collection
- Flowchart

U (Understand the Problem and the Causes of Process Variation)

Variation occurs in any process, however controlled it seems to be. One key to improving quality is to reduce variation, which in turn improves reliability. Knowing the type of variation is helpful in managing continuous improvement. The purpose of this section is to determine which factors in the process cause variation and, if they are changed, may improve the quality characteristics defined for the process.

In this step of the improvement process, the team should determine which factors (manpower, machines, materials, methods, environment, and measurements) cause variation in the outcome of the process (process variables). Which of these, if changed, would improve the outcome of the KQCs? These are the KPVs. This is best done with a cause-and-effect diagram. Pareto and scatter charts may be of value in proving which is the most important and indicating the relationships between the KPVs and KQCs (Figures 4.5, 4.6, and 4.7).

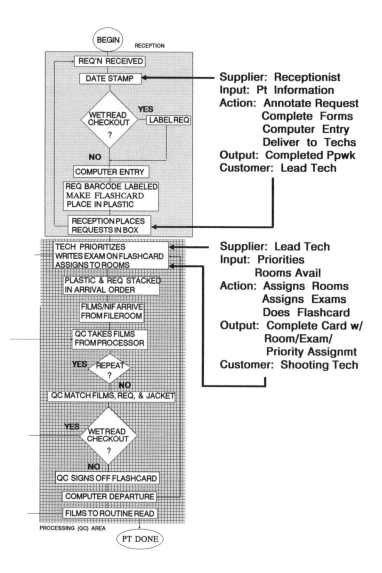

Figure 4.4 Assigning Process to the Flowchart

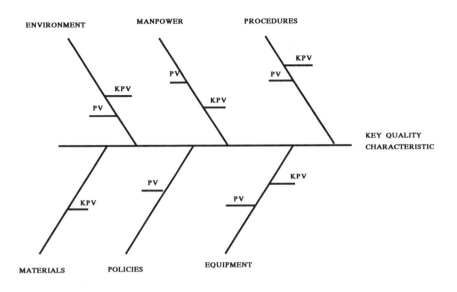

Figure 4.5 Fishbone Diagram of Cause and Effect

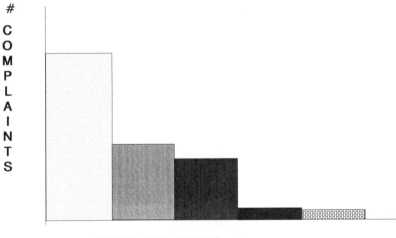

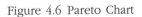

Figure 4.6 Pareto Chart

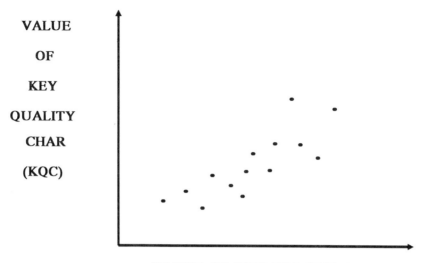

Figure 4.7 Scatter Diagram

Tools commonly employed in identifying variation and its effect on quality include:

- Brainstorming
- Data collection
- Pareto chart
- Cause-and-effect diagram (fishbone chart)
- Stratification
- Histogram
- Trend (run) chart
- Control chart

S (Select the Method to Improve the Process)

Having identified the major process variables (KPVs) that have the greatest effect on the outcome (KQC), what can be done to improve the outcome? Propose several solutions and study the impact and side effects of each proposed change on the entire process. Also, evaluate the improvement with an eye to the opportunity statement and the vision, mission, and guiding principles of the organization.

An obvious improvement may already have come to mind. There is no reason to delay implementing such an idea. However, ensure that this "obvious improvement" fits the following criteria:

- Everyone on the team must agree that the improvement is obvious.
- The improvement should not adversely affect any other process.
- The improvement should not require the supplier or customer of the process to change what they are currently doing.

Use PDCA to implement and evaluate the change.

Tools commonly employed in selecting the improvement include:

- Brainstorming
- Data collection
- Pareto charts
- Graphs and charts
- Stratification

P (Plan to Implement the New Method and Measure the Change)

The plan should include (1) clear objectives and goals, (2) the steps for implementation including training of personnel involved, (3) assumptions made in the absence of data and contingency plans in case the assumptions are wrong, and (4) measurements that will guide the analysis of the effect of the change.

Do not underestimate the power of workers in implementing change, if they are included in the process.

Tools commonly employed in planning the change include:

- Brainstorming
- Flowchart
- Cause-and-effect diagram

D (Do the Implementation and Measurement)

Educate the people involved in the change. Train them to do things differently and make sure they understand why the change is necessary. The basic goals, policies, and standards that are being applied must be communicated to the people responsible for carrying out the change. The success of this step will determine the success of the implementation.

Put the change into effect. Is the change being effectively carried out? Are data being obtained?

Tools commonly employed in implementing the change include:

- Pareto chart
- Flowchart

- Graphs and charts
- Histogram
- Trend (run) chart
- Control chart

C (Check the Results of the Change)

Checking activities can be divided into causes and effects. Causes of variations must be identified during and after the change. Some causes of adverse outcomes or problems in the process will show weaknesses in the standards set for the change. These must be actively identified by management. A checklist of causes (process variables) from a fishbone diagram may be helpful.

Included in the plan for implementation must be a method for measuring the effects of the change. This requires baseline information, which can be obtained from pilot studies. These effects must be immediately communicated to the workers involved in the process.

Tools commonly employed in following up on the results of the change include:

- Data collection
- Pareto chart
- Flowchart
- Cause-and-effect diagram
- Graphs and charts
- Stratification
- Histogram
- Trend (run) chart
- Control chart

A (Act to Hold the Improvements and Continue Further Improvements)

Expand the improvements and knowledge of the improved processes. Identify the next most important problem to solve and apply FOCUS-PDCA.

Tools commonly employed to maintain continuous improvement include:

- Brainstorming
- Data collection
- Pareto chart
- Cause-and-effect diagram
- Graphs and charts
- Stratification

TOTAL QUALITY IMPROVEMENT
IMPLEMENTATION PLAN

The following steps in problem solving and continuous improvement assume a working knowledge of the Deming Management Method. Newly formed Quality Improvement Teams may need additional familiarization with this method in order to carry out their tasks. This is the purpose of the following implementation plan. Each step includes references to chapters in this book that should be reviewed with participants prior to undertaking the task.

1. Find an area you want to improve (F) (Chapters 3 and 5).
2. Introduce Deming's 14 points and the concepts of TQM (Chapter 1).
   Task: Discuss the points as they apply to the practice and encourage free discussion.
3. Introduce TQM (Chapters 1 and 2).
   Task: Define a vision and mission for the practice or organization. Adopt guiding principles as needed. Are they consistent with the statements of the parent organization (if any)?
4. Review process definition and FOCUS-PDCA (Chapters 3 and 4).
   Task: Draft and review an opportunity statement (F). Is it consistent with the vision, mission, and guiding principles? Organize a team. Is the team appropriate to study the problem (O) and consistent with the opportunity statement?
5. Review the basic process of supplier, input, action, output, customer, and needs/expectations (Chapter 3). Review flowcharting, KQCs, and the seven basic tools of total quality improvement (Chapter 5).
   Task: Clarify the process with a flowchart (C). Determine the basic subprocesses that make up the entire flowchart. Define the KQCs. Verify that the opportunity statement, team membership, and clarification of the problem are in alignment and consistent with the vision, mission, and guiding principles.
6. Review understanding of the problem and variation (cause-and-effect chart, KPVs, and data collection (U). Introduce basic statistics (Chapter 6) and apply the seven tools (Chapter 5). These simple tools are the basis for performing total quality improvement. They must be mastered in order to proceed further with success.
   Task: Construct a cause-and-effect diagram for each basic process. Define the KPVs. Define data collection necessary for fact finding. Verify alignment of **F, O, C,** and **U** and consistency with the vision, mission, and guiding principles.

7. *Task:* Collect data as necessary to further understand the problem issues.
8. Review Select (**S**) and select data as appropriate.
    Task: Apply data to appropriate charts. Select changes necessary to improve the process (**S**). Check alignment of FOCUS and consistency.
9. Review Plan (**P**).
    Task: Plan to implement the improvement and continue data collection (**P**). Determine goals and targets and methods for achieving them.
10. Review Do (**D**).
    Task: Engage in education and training for the proposed improvement and try it out (**D**).
11. Review Check (**C**).
    Task: Check the results and lessons learned from the attempt (**C**).
12. Review Act (**A**).
    Task: Act to hold the gains and continue to improve the process (**A**) such that replacing any of the team members will not disrupt the continuity of improvement.

5

MASTERING
the TOOLS of TQM

Workers must master the tools of the job.

Kaoru Ishikawa

Over the years, statistical methods and tools have become as much an integral part of TQM in various manufacturing and service industries as the teamwork needed to apply them. To a limited degree, these tools have been used in quality control and quality audits in the healthcare industry.

Statistical tools are useful in the design, implementation, and maintenance phases of TQM. When correctly used, these tools facilitate accurate interpretation of facts. Busy practitioners of radiology are not expected to master all the statistical techniques; however, a working knowledge of these basic statistical tools will be helpful in tackling various clinical quality problems in the practice. Radiology managers can use these tools to evaluate working conditions and costs, identify and prioritize problems to be addressed, etc.

Seven basic statistical tools serve as communication devices:

1. Flowchart
2. Cause-and-effect diagram
3. Histogram
4. Pareto chart
5. Scatter diagram
6. Trend chart
7. Control chart

The following tools improve group dynamics as well:

1. Brainstorming
2. Multivoting
3. Nominal group technique
4. Consensus

FLOWCHART

A flowchart is a visual outline of all the actions in a process. It depicts the relationship among various steps in a process and is helpful in identifying sites of possible system failure, waste, or improvement. Examples of flowcharts are provided in Figures 5.1A and 5.1B.

Rules to follow in flowcharting include:

1. Identify inputs, actions, and outputs and chart them as they currently exist.
2. Start with a rough guide of how each process works and then draft a more detailed view, specifying each step.
3. Chart each area in which additional work is created by not completing the action properly.
4. Do not exceed the boundaries that determine what is being studied.
5. Leave no blind limbs. Each pathway must tie into another part of the flowchart or must represent the end of a process.

Standard Symbols for Flowcharts

The activity symbol in a flowchart is a rectangle. A brief description of that activity is contained within the rectangle.

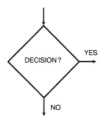

The decision symbol is a diamond. It designates a decision point

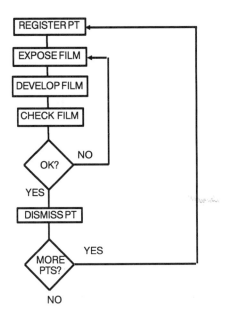

Figure 5.1A Patient Throughput Flowchart

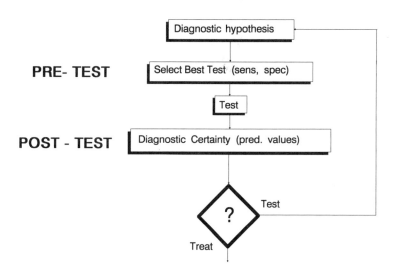

Figure 5.1B Flowchart of Diagnostic Decision Pathway

from which the process branches into two or more paths. Each path corresponds to an answer to the question within the diamond. A decision point with more than three pathways leading from it may be represented by a hexagon, octagon, etc.

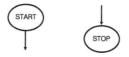

The terminal symbol is a rounded rectangle or an oval. It identifies the beginning or the end of a process.

The flow line represents a path which connects process elements. The arrowhead on a flow line indicates the direction of flow of the process.

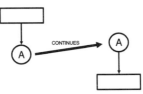

The connector is a circle. It is used to indicate a continuation of the flow diagram.

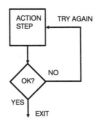

Loops are circuitous pathways that may represent frequently re-peated steps, rework loops, or feedback loops. There must be at least one decision point in each loop in order to exit the loop.

Macro vs. Micro Flowcharts

In the beginning of an improvement process, it may be helpful to flowchart the overall schema (macro flowchart) and examine the major

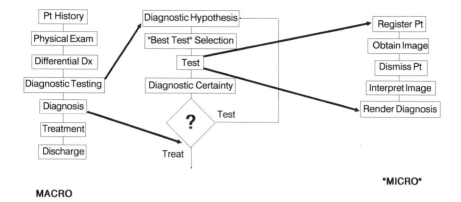

MACRO   **"MICRO"**

Figure 5.2 Macro Flowchart vs. Micro Flowchart

steps. This helps determine the major suppliers, inputs, actions, outputs, and customers.

A macro flowchart is useful in defining the process variables that arise from the suppliers, inputs, and actions. In addition, the quality characteristics of the outputs and the needs and expectations of the customers can be identified.

When further understanding of the process is needed, a micro flowchart may be of assistance. The micro flowchart is more detailed than the macro flowchart and identifies further opportunities for improvement (Figure 5.2).

CAUSE-AND-EFFECT DIAGRAM

This graphic tool is also called a fishbone chart (because of its obvious appearance) or an Ishikawa diagram (named for the person who devised it). It is a problem-solving tool which graphically demonstrates causes and effects (Figure 5.3). It is used to illustrate various causes (process variables) that affect a given key quality characteristic and to create starting points for determining the key process variables.

After identifying the variables that affect the key quality characteristic, each can be measured to determine which is the most important. When the most important variable is minimized by good problem solving, the next most important variable is addressed, thereby producing continuous improvement.

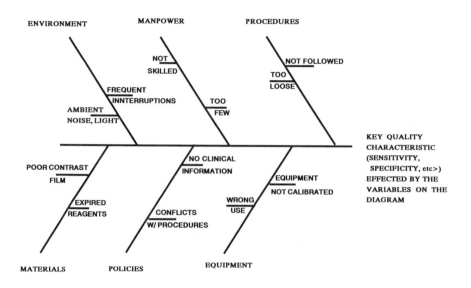

Figure 5.3 Fishbone Diagram of Cause and Effect

The cause-and-effect or fishbone diagram graphically demonstrates those variables that influence a measurable quality. Brainstorming is a useful technique to identify such causes as manpower, policies, procedures, environment, equipment, and materials. The relationship between the variable and the quality characteristic can be determined by using a scatter diagram.

The following is an example of causes which influence the sensitivity or specificity of diagnostic examinations. An improper examination method may adversely affect the ability of the study to detect an abnormality, such as using a 10-mm slice thickness on CT or MRI to evaluate the IAC. An improper reading environment may distract the radiologist, resulting in failure to detect disease. Using high-density barium for "solid column" BEs will likely decrease the ability to detect small polyps.

HISTOGRAM

A histogram is a bar graph (Figure 5.4). The height of each bar on the vertical axis (ordinate) represents either the absolute or relative frequency of the categories (class interval) shown on the horizontal axis (abscissa). It is easy to construct and interpret. Analysis of dispersion

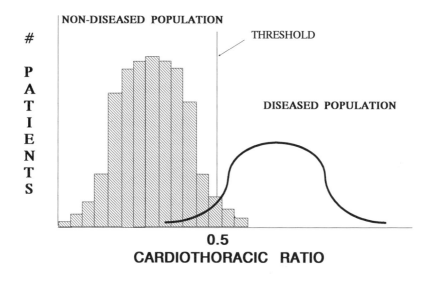

Figure 5.4 Sample Histogram

shape, center value, and nature of dispersion is helpful in revealing problems. A histogram identifies the amount of variation within a process.

A histogram is a graphic display of frequency of occurrence. It is useful in further understanding the operations and in decision making. An example might be the number of walk-in patients presenting during a given time frame, to assist in defining staffing requirements during the day. Another example is the distribution of patients displaying certain diagnostic criteria, such as the cardiothoracic ratio in a population of patients with and without heart disease.

PARETO CHART

This chart is named after Wilfredo Pareto, an Italian political economist, who used a variation of the histogram to demonstrate that a large portion of the wealth in his country was controlled by a very small portion of the population.

The Pareto chart is diagrammatic representation of the Pareto principle (introduced by Juran), which states that a few causes typically account for most of the problems and other causes are generally less important. The Pareto chart is a column graph with the highest priority

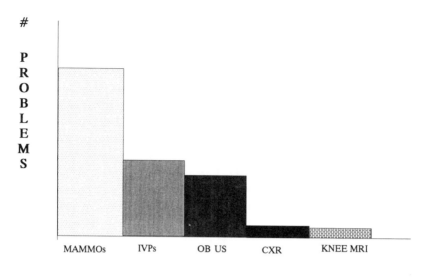

Figure 5.5 Pareto Chart

problem on the left and the other problems in decreasing order to the right (Figure 5.5). A Pareto chart is useful in selecting projects for improvement (by priority) and identifying the main causes of problems.

SCATTER DIAGRAM

The scatter diagram shows the relationship between the key process variables and the key quality characteristics (Figure 5.6A). In a scatter diagram, each of the *n* pairs (X_i, Y_i) is plotted as a single point, with *X* values plotted on the horizontal axis (abscissa) and *Y* values plotted on the vertical axis (ordinate).

If a large *X* value coincides with a large *Y* value and a small *X* value coincides with a small *Y* value, the relationship between *X* and *Y* is positive. If a large *X* value corresponds with a small *Y* value and vice versa, the relationship is negative.

The example in Figure 5.6B illustrates the well-known positive relationship between diagnostic ability and the number of exams performed annually.

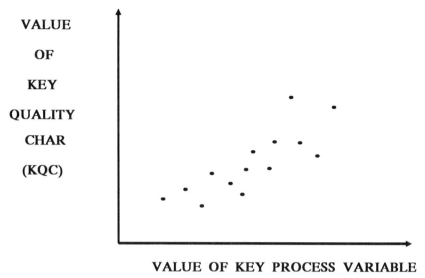

VALUE
OF
KEY
QUALITY
CHAR
(KQC)

**VALUE OF KEY PROCESS VARIABLE
(KPV)**

Figure 5.6A Scatter Diagram

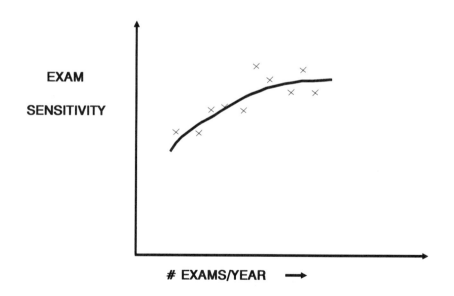

**EXAM
SENSITIVITY**

 # EXAMS/YEAR ➝

Figure 5.6B Scatter Diagram

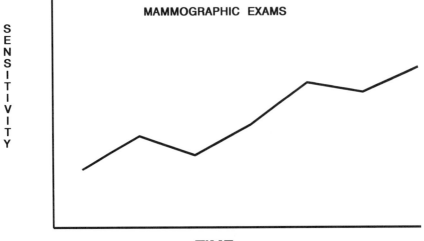

Figure 5.7 Trend Chart

TREND CHART

Also called a run chart, a trend chart visually represents data to determine whether key indicators are moving up or down (e.g., increasing or decreasing) and whether that is good or bad. It is used to monitor a system in order to determine whether or not the long-range average is changing.

A trend chart is a simpler version of a control chart. Unlike the latter, however, it does not identify conditions that are under control or out of control. Thus, it does not indicate when corrective action is required.

A trend chart is a graphic display of measurements as a function of time. The example in Figure 5.7 indicates improvement in the sensitivity of mammographic interpretations over time, such as might be expected in a practice employing a quality improvement program.

CONTROL CHART

A control chart displays the performance of a process over time and is used to determine whether that process is consistent and operating in statistical control. The chart consists of three lines. The center line is obtained by averaging the value of 20 to 25 sample statistics. It is usually a measure of some characteristic that is key to the quality of the operation. The upper and lower lines (control limits) represent the limits within which the values of the statistics should fall with a specified probability. In quality control situations, this range of control limits is usually determined by plus or minus three standard deviations.

The two main types of control charts are the attribute control chart and the variables control chart. Attribute control charts are constructed by counting the number of items in one of two categories. The categories represent the presence or absence of the characteristic being examined. This chart is especially useful in analyzing productivity, efficiency, improvement of backlog, and other areas affected by manpower.

Variables control charts are based on numerical measurements. They provide specific data about a single characteristic of a process and provide clues to help isolate the problem. When the value exceeds the upper or lower control limit, intervention must take place to determine the cause and correct it.

In order to completely evaluate a process, sampling should occur at times when changes occur in the process (i.e., changes in manpower, shift changes, etc.). Rational subgroups should be defined so that changes in results between groups can provide an indication of the cause. If a chart shows increasing or decreasing trends, the process should be investigated to determine the cause before the control limits are exceeded.

Recall that the purpose of continuous improvement is to improve the quality characteristic (central line) and minimize the variation (control limits) around it. Examples of quality characteristics include patient waiting time, sensitivity, specificity, or predictive value of an exam. In controlled systems the actual measured value will normally vary around the central line. When the value exceeds the upper or lower control limit, intervention must take place to determine the causeand correct it.

In Figure 5.8, the central line may be the monthly complication rate for procedures done in the practice. The upper and lower control limits can be as reported in the literature or can be calculated based on data from the practice. The lines plotted above and below the central line may be the complication rates for individual providers. While the QA approach in the past may have been to fire the provider with the higher rate, TQM differs in two respects: (1) it studies why one provider has a lower rate and (2) it applies what is learned from this provider to the other provider(s) for improvement. By improving the ability of providers

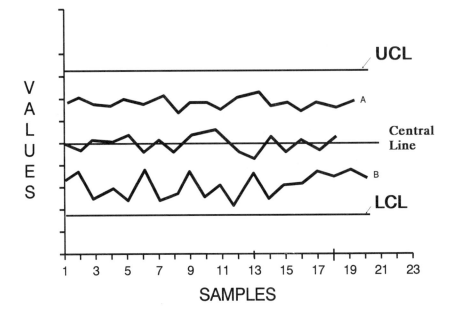

Figure 5.8 Quality Control Chart

with higher rates, the rate throughout the practice is improved. Variation between providers is narrowed, and the quality of the practice is improved.

GROUP TASK AND DECISION-MAKING TOOLS

Much of the work in total quality improvement is conducted by groups of people dedicated to the idea that the processes for which they are responsible can continually be improved. Some of the methods used to make decisions and reach agreement within these groups are reviewed in the following sections. These methods include brainstorming, multivoting, consensus, rank ordering, and nominal group technique.

Brainstorming

Webster's New World Dictionary defines brainstorming as "the unrestrained offering of ideas or suggestions by all members of a group meeting." The purpose behind such a device is to generate a large number of ideas from all members of the team for the purpose of exploring reasonable options to be considered in the decision-making process.

The leader of a brainstorming session should encourage everyone to participate (drawing out those hesitant to say anything), encourage free discussion while maintaining relevance to the issue at hand, build on the ideas of others, and record all of the ideas generated.

Several caveats in leading a brainstorming session include not criticizing any contribution in order to eliminate fear of censure, recording all ideas including those that may be a subset or superset of another idea already recorded, and cutting off discussion as to the merit of an idea.

Several steps can be used to conduct a brainstorming session:

1. Inform team members of the topic prior to the session.
2. Review the subject to be addressed during the meeting.
3. Pose the issue to be discussed in the form of a question.
4. Take turns offering ideas that address the topic at hand or split into small groups to facilitate the flow of ideas.
5. Record all ideas.
6. Encourage members to expand on the ideas of others.
7. Consolidate related thoughts.

Once the comprehensive list of items has been consolidated and agreed upon, some sense of order or priority should be applied. This is accomplished by using the next three group activity tools: consensus, multivoting, and rank ordering.

Consensus

In making a decision, the team must reach some agreement as to the best course of action from among the options identified. This agreement is known as consensus and is defined as that which the members find sufficiently acceptable to support the actions that follow the decision. It does not require total agreement or unanimous approval, but it must be acceptable to each member.

In reaching consensus, each member is allowed to state his or her position regarding the issue at hand. Time will be required to listen, identify conflicts or opposing positions, and encourage discussion. An open-minded atmosphere must prevail. Creative thinking is essential.

Multivoting

After exploring numerous options or issues, multivoting is used to weed out the more superfluous items in order to concentrate on the most important ones. This can be accomplished by listing and numbering all the options or issues, allowing all members to vote for up to one third of the issues they believe to be most important, tabulating the votes and eliminating those items with the fewest votes, and repeating the process until only a few items remain.

The issue or decision can be selected from among those with the most votes or one last poll may be necessary to determine which is considered to be most important.

Rank Ordering

This is similar to multivoting in that a large list of items can be reduced to those that are most pressing (according to the members). Each idea on the list is identified by a letter. Each member ranks all or a portion (n) of the list (1 = most important, n = least important). The rank order numbers for each item are recorded and totaled. The item with the smallest number would be considered the most important.

Nominal Group Technique

This is a more structured technique than those discussed previously. It is useful in situations where the group is large or the members are unfamiliar with one another.

It begins with the leader distributing a sheet of paper on which the issue before the group is posed as a question. Each member is asked to list his or her ideas in writing. No discussion or distractions should be allowed.

Once everyone has finished, each member reads his or her ideas, which are then listed on a flip chart. No discussion should be allowed. When the list is complete, clarification and discussion can ensue to focus the idea or amend the wording. Only the person who proposed the idea can approve a change in wording.

In order to narrow the list, a technique similar to multivoting can be used or the technique can be more highly structured, such as giving a proportion of the items on the list a point value and tallying the results. Issues with the highest point value will likely represent those most in need of attention. If members agree that the item that received the highest point total is the most important, then the discussion is over. If members disagree, then discussion should focus on those items with the highest point totals before voting again.

SUMMARY

The preceding discussion described basic statistical tools that are helpful in distinguishing variation in quality due to chance causes, where no intervention is required, and variation due to specific causes, which offers an opportunity to improve the process.

A Pareto chart, trend chart, or histogram may be used to identify where and when a problem occurs and to state the extent of problem. A flowchart and Pareto chart are ideal tools for prioritizing problems. A Pareto chart, histogram, or control chart may be used to implement and monitor the solutions established. Group techniques improve the effectiveness of the team in processing information and making decisions.

6

The BASICS of
STATISTICAL ANALYSIS

...we measure as the basis for future improvement.

Dennis S. O'Leary, M.D.
Preface to *The Measurement Mandate*
JCAHO

DOING IT WITH DATA

Recall from the previous chapters that Total Quality Management (TQM) is a structured problem-solving process that uses statistical means to produce better long-term solutions than would be produced by unstructured wild guesses or even educated guesses. The purpose of this chapter is to review basic statistics for the administrator, worker, or physician who wants to apply quality improvement in his or her practice.

It has been said many times that any lie can be proven to be a truth by using statistics. This is, of course, an exaggeration and results from the misuse or misunderstanding of numbers. We hope to provide the reader with an appreciation of the correct use of statistics in support of the improvement of quality in the practice of radiology.

Chapter 5 provided a detailed discussion of the basic tools of TQM. The successful employment of many of these graphic tools requires the use of information, facts, and data to support and, in some cases, construct them. Even in selecting which problem should be addressed first, data may be needed to determine which situation is most vital to improving or maintaining the practice. When measuring the key quality characteristics or identifying the causes of variability in measuring them, data collection will likely be necessary to (1) address the most important (recall the 80/20 rule) and (2) test the theories of cause and effect.

In planning for data collection, it is important to consider the following:

1. What information is needed or what questions need to be answered?
2. What TQM tools are needed, and what data are needed to apply these tools?
3. Where in the process can the data be found?
4. How can the data be collected with a minimum of effort and error?
5. What additional information may be needed after the initial questions have been answered? Can data that may answer future questions be captured at the same time?
6. How much data is needed to provide a reasonably accurate description of the entire "population" in question?

The first five points are left to the reader's careful consideration at the time of implementation. Because of the cost of data collection, the last point is discussed in detail in this chapter (see Sampling).

BASIC DESCRIPTIVE STATISTICS

Understanding the basics of statistics is essential for participating in total quality improvement. It has repeatedly been said that certain tools must be mastered and applied daily in order for continuous improvement to work. In Japan, these principles are learned by almost the entire work force, most of whom have at least a high school education. The American work force is equally capable of understanding the concepts and their applications. The future of the healthcare industry may depend on learning and applying these simple concepts.

This brief overview is intended to provide the statistical tools necessary to collect the data needed to identify opportunities for improvement. The tools to be mastered include the concept of groups of items to be measured (*populations, samples, data sets*) and the mathematic operations needed to reduce the data to useful information that is representative of the group being measured (*frequency, maximum, minimum, mean, median, mode,* and *standard deviation*).

Populations

Obviously, population in this context is not a census count of citizens. *Population* in statistical terms refers to the entire group or set of items being measured. The first task in obtaining data for total quality improvement is to identify the population or set of items to be measured. In X-ray, the population set may be the patients examined during a month or the number of phone calls received. It is important to specify what aspect of the group in question is to be measured (i.e., waiting time for patients or the type of phone calls received).

In most cases, when large numbers are being considered, it is not practical to measure every item; rather, a small number within the population is measured. The number of items that are actually measured from a set or population is known as a representative *sample* and as such is a chosen proportion, or subset, of the population. For example, we may measure something about every fifth or twentieth patient or every other exam. In the first case, 20% of the population would be measured, 5% in the second case, and 50% in the third case. (How to choose an appropriate sample size will be addressed later.)

The measurements obtained are known collectively as the *data set*. The data set may provide information that would not likely be predicted with any great certainty in advance. The results are inferred to represent the entire population and are thus a *statistical inference*. The objective of the measurement is to use the information obtained from the representative sample to infer what is likely taking place in the entire population. This will be covered in greater detail in the following sections.

Data Description

Once the data set has been obtained, it must be displayed in such a way that it is useful. The data set can be displayed graphically as the *frequency* of occurrence in the set (histogram) or numerically by reducing the data set to values of *maximum, minimum, mean* (average), *median, mode,* and *standard deviation*. How we use the data is determined by what we need to know.

Frequency

In determining the frequency of observation, the number of observations in each defined category is counted. One example is the number of patients examined in X-ray in the categories walk-in, emergency room patients, inpatients, etc. Another example is the distribution of waiting times at intervals of 0 to 10 minutes, 11 to 20 minutes, and 21 to 30 minutes or the number of patients that presented for examination categorized by the time of day they arrived.

To illustrate frequency, the number of patients who experienced waiting times in categories of 10-minute intervals is recorded in Table 6.1. A frequency plot (histogram) of this data set is presented in Figure 6.1. This frequency distribution shows that the majority of patients were examined in less than an hour. However, one patient waited for more than 150 minutes.

The data provide an opportunity for detailed examination of those patients outside the norm in order to determine why they waited so long and to correct the cause of the variation (the reason for the lengthy wait). At the other end of the spectrum, it may be meaningful to study those patients who experienced a brief stay in the department and use this information to improve waiting times for all patients.

Mode

The mode is the measurement that occurs most often. In our example, the mode was 21 to 30 minutes.

Maximum

The maximum is the largest observed value in the data set. In our example, the maximum was 155 minutes.

Minimum

The minimum is the smallest observed value in the data set. In our example, the minimum waiting time observed was 9 minutes.

Mean

Also known as the average of a set of observations, the mean is simply the sum of the observed values divided by the number of observations. This value reduces the data set to one number which is the arithmetic middle of the road. In our example of waiting time, the mean was 41.6 minutes:

Computation example:

$$\text{Data set: } 2, \ 4, \ 2, \ 6, \ 2, \ 1, \ 4$$

$$\text{Mean}: \quad \frac{2 + 4 + 2 + 6 + 2 + 1 + 4}{7} = 3$$

Table 6.1 Patient Waiting Time Frequencies

Waiting time	Frequency	Mean	Standard deviation
0–10	1	41.60	25.55
11–20	28		
21–30	40		
31–40	23		
41–50	24		
51–60	17		
61–70	8		
71–80	7		
81–90	5		
91–100	0		
101–110	3		
111–120	0		
121–130	1		
131–140	1		
141–150	0		
151–160	1		
161–180	0		
181–200	0		
201–300	0		

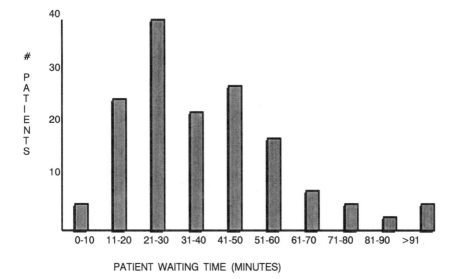

Figure 6.1 Histogram of Patient Waiting Time Frequencies

Median

The mean should not be confused with the median, which is the event which has an equal number of observations less than and more than its value. The median is the numeric middle:

Data set:	2, 2, 4, 6, 2, 1, 4
Ordered data set:	1, 2, 2, **2**, 4, 4, 6
Median = 2	

Standard Deviation

This value demonstrates the variation of events around the mean. The standard deviation is usually applied as the range surrounding the mean (the value of the mean plus or minus the standard deviation). The range of values included in the range of plus or minus one standard deviation contains approximately 68% of the total number of observations in the data set. Approximately 95% of the total observations in the data set lie within two standard deviations. Over 99% of the observations lie within three standard deviations of the mean.

Data set: 2, 4, 2, 6, 2, 1, 4

Standard deviation :

$$= \frac{[(3-2)^2 + (3-4)^2 + (3-2)^2 + (3-6)^2 + (3-2)^2 + (3-1)^2 + (3-4)^2]^{1/2}}{7^{1/2}}$$
$$= 1.60$$

When large variation occurs, three possible factors must be considered: (1) this may be normal, (2) something may be wrong with the way the measurements were defined or obtained (i.e., the measuring procedure included both angiograms and fluoro studies with the walk-in exams), or (3) the system may be out of control. The purpose of total quality improvement is to minimize the variation and thereby reduce the standard deviation.

Industry usually considers three standard deviations as the range of interest so as to include over 99% of the total observations. It is this range that we want to reduce by reducing the variability.

In our example of waiting time, the standard deviation was 25.55 minutes, indicating that 68% of the patients in the sample waited from 15 to 67.1 minutes. If the standard deviation is near 100 minutes, there is probably too much variability. We are interested in reducing the average waiting time as well as the range of waiting times.

Sampling

Measurements are observations that define the behavior of the characteristics of the process (i.e., waiting time, repeat rate, sensitivity, etc.). It will be helpful to define the type of numerical variables (as differentiated from process variable) being measured in order to understand the following applications.

Continuous variables arise from an infinite arithmetic scale of values. Examples include time, weight, age, etc. *Dichotomous variables* are those that have only two values or choices (i.e., the presence or absence of disease, on/off, male/female). Continuous variables are most often applied in the statistics of departmental logistics. Dichotomous variables are most frequently applied in diagnostic science.

The key to sampling is to know when and how much to sample in order to provide fairly accurate inferences. For example, suppose that the X-ray department examines 4000 walk-in patients monthly and only two are sampled by measuring their waiting times. What if these two people happen to wait an excessive period of time? This is probably not a good measure of the average waiting time for most patients.

Conversely, what if the two happen to easily transit the department. Is it correct to infer that all 4000 patients met the same fate? However, 5% or 200 patients randomly sampled and measured may provide a more accurate presentation of the average waiting time for the entire group.

An even more accurate value could be obtained by sampling 50% of the patients, but at this sampling rate the measuring task may become overwhelming and expensive. What level of accuracy and precision is necessary? The answer will of course depend upon the circumstances. A very high level of accuracy is required in diagnostic treatment decisions, while a lower level of accuracy is probably acceptable in measuring logistics.

Sampling Frequency vs. Accuracy

In sampling, we are attempting to describe what is happening with our entire population by measuring what happens to a smaller subset of the whole. How many samples we must take depends on how much accuracy we desire. We must decide how close we want our result to be to the actual value and how much confidence we want in the result.

Just like the political polls heard on the evening news, there is always a margin of error in the results unless the entire population is sampled. In general, the larger the sample size the more accurate the results. But how much is too much sampling? What can the organization afford? For logistic decision making we have used 200–250 samples over the examination period to provide reasonable guidance. For diagnostic and therapeutic decision making the statistical design should reflect consideration of the costs of type I and type II errors.

For critical decision making we recommend consulting a text on biomedical statistics or a statistician. An adequate discussion of sampling is beyond the scope of this text. We expect to discuss this topic at length in another text of advanced quality improvement.

BASIC STATISTICS OF DIAGNOSIS

Diagnostic testing has been the boon and the bane of healthcare during this century. It has improved our ability to diagnose and provide therapy in a more timely manner, but it has also increased the cost of care considerably. This cost and the burgeoning array of examinations and tests that compete for a share of the healthcare dollar have prompted public officials and corporate executives to call for closer scrutiny of expenditures for diagnostic testing and for improvements in diagnostic capabilities.

Diagnostic improvements have usually been relegated to university programs, but even these institutions have not always withstood comparative measures of effectiveness in the cost of diagnosing and treating certain diagnosis-related groupings (DRGs). Can most of us say that we have compared our diagnostic capabilities against a standard and exceeded it? Do such standards exist? Moreover, does Quality Assurance (QA) provide for improved care?

The shortcomings of QA are well known. It established the concepts of identifying provider-specific problems and meeting literature-supported standards. The premise was that if the standards were met, any problems that existed were caused by factors outside of the system, and a provider could be identified as the source. Little attention was paid to the support systems which influenced the care provided or to extenuating circumstances. The "bad apple" was to be found and eliminated.

Another shortcoming of QA was the standards-driven focus of retrospective examination. This is certainly a reasonable approach to "assuring" the quality of what has already been provided, but it reveals little about what must be done to improve. A major premise of TQM, on the other hand, is that quality must be built in from the ground up.

The Agenda for Change presented by the Joint Commission for Accreditation of Healthcare Organizations (JCAHO) is a remarkable shift in focus from meeting standards toward the concept of implementing continuous improvement. This shift provides the opportunity to "assure" the quality of diagnostic testing by building quality into the test or examination as it is produced, rather than after it has been completed. In addition, a built-in mechanism is provided to continuously improve the exam or test by repeatedly improving the "standard," which may ultimately result in improved diagnosis and decreased cost.

Such an undertaking requires an appropriate definition of quality as well as the diagnostic process in order to identify areas for improvement and to quantify the diagnostic product. Dr. David Eddy, one of the leaders in healthcare today, indicates that quality in medical care is determined by two factors: (1) the quality of the *decisions* that determine what actions are taken and (2) the quality with which those actions are carried out. Evaluating the actions is the same as logistics. However, evaluating the decision-making process requires a model to which the tools of continuous quality improvement can be applied. A diagnostic model is proposed in the next section, followed by a discussion of its application to quality improvement.

The Diagnostic Model

In order to measure the patient's clinical encounter, it must first be modeled, as follows:

- **Pre-test**
  Patient history obtained
  Physical examination conducted
  Possible diagnoses entertained
  Selection of diagnostic testing as necessary

- **Post-test**
  Analysis of results
  Diagnosis
  Treatment
  Follow-up
  Discharge

This model is divided into pre-test and post-test diagnostic phases in order to facilitate the discussion. It should be understood that diagnostic testing and analysis is a continuous loop which can be exited in the flow of this model only when sufficient diagnostic certainty is achieved (Figure 6.2).

It is important for physicians to distinguish between the pre- and post-test phases of medical diagnosis. The pre-test phase refers to that part of the process which hypothesizes that the patient has a disease and

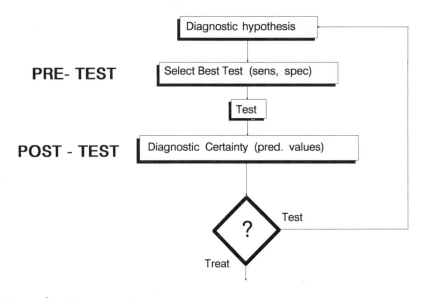

Figure 6.2 Diagnostic Testing Loop

projects the pre-test likelihood that the proposed exam will detect it or rule it out with some degree of certainty. In essence, the physician is requesting an exam of sufficient sensitivity to detect the disease which the patient is proposed to have and of sufficient specificity to differentiate the disease from other masquerading pathology.

The post-test phase of diagnosis refers to that part of the process which yields information to improve the physician's certainty about the diagnosis (predictive value). The intent in diagnostic testing is, of course, to maximize the diagnostic certainty prior to instituting therapy. The cost and risk of each test must be taken into consideration in deciding whether to treat or continue testing as the diagnostic curve moves toward certainty (Figure 6.3). In terms of quality improvement, anything that can be done to improve the certainty, decrease the time to diagnosis, or reduce the number of exams will improve patient care and may decrease costs.

Cases that are easily diagnosed have a curve that rapidly approaches certainty with a minimum of diagnostic testing. More difficult cases require more extensive testing to reach a level of certainty to allow therapy to begin.

It is well known that diagnostic tests are less than perfect. Because diseased and non-diseased populations vary in their physiologic or pathologic means and overlap to some extent (Figure 6.4), the false negatives and false positives which this type of testing and examination

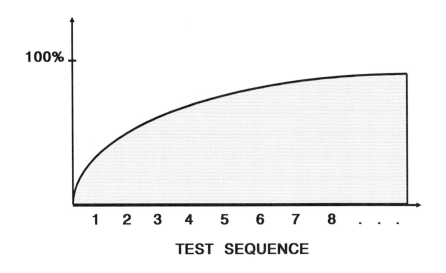

Figure 6.3 Diagnostic Certainty Curve

yields represents a problem. Diagnosis necessitates that positive and negative results in testing be defined; thus, a threshold must be established above or below which a test can be defined as positive. The value of the test to diagnosticians depends on choosing a threshold such that false positives and false negatives are minimized. In the clinical laboratory, this may be the value of a serum concentration; in radiology, it may be the presence or absence of certain radiographic characteristics.

If one attribute of healthcare quality can be defined as the capability of diagnostic examinations, a model can be constructed to facilitate its improvement. The underlying goal in this analysis is to identify quantitative methods to measure the capability or quality of diagnostic exams.

The Measure of Quality in Diagnostic Tests

Defining quality in medicine is not an easy task. To facilitate definition, one might consider that every model of service has a supplier and a customer. Quality is usually defined by the knowledgeable customer in such settings as meeting or exceeding the customer's needs and expectations. However, in medicine some knowledge is not easily obtainable by the average patient (customer). It is in these circumstances that the physician has a fiduciary responsibility to define those aspects of medical quality that are unknown to the patient. Selecting the appropriate test and maximizing the accurate interpretation of the results

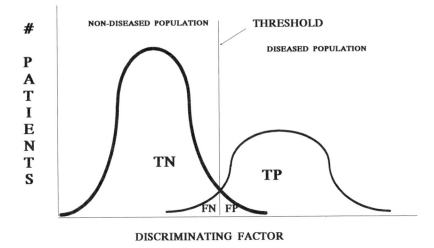

Figure 6.4 Diseased and Non-Diseased Populations

are examples of qualities that a patient may not be able to articulate but nevertheless desires.

Obtaining the appropriate test and analyzing the results of the exam requires an understanding of the statistics of diagnosis. This entails little more than a working knowledge of a results table and an appreciation of the proportions of diseased and non-diseased populations. The results table in Figure 6.5 is a representation of a binary test [one that has either a positive (+) or negative (−) result].

Evaluation of the Pre-Test Capability

The measurable values in assessing exam pre-test capability are as follows.

- **Sensitivity** (also known as pre-test true positive rate): TP/(TP + FN). The likelihood of obtaining a positive test in a patient with disease.
- **Specificity** (also known as pre-test true negative rate): TN/(TN + FP). The likelihood of obtaining a negative test in a patient without disease.
- **Pre-test false-negative rate** (1 − sensitivity): The likelihood of obtaining a negative test in a patient with disease.
- **Pre-test false positive rate** (1 − specificity): The likelihood of obtaining a positive test in a patient without disease.

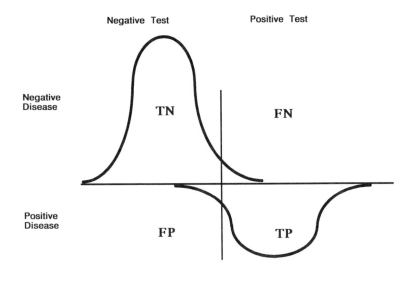

Figure 6.5 Results Table

These definitions are examples of likelihoods or probabilities that have preconditions, i.e., conditional probabilities. Thus, the pre-test condition is the hypothesized presence or absence of disease in a patient, and the probability is the likelihood of a particular test outcome given the condition of the presence or absence of disease.

The following question is asked in the testing phase of diagnostic imaging: "If a patient has disease X, what is the likelihood of test Y being positive?" This probability is defined as the sensitivity of the test. For a pre-test condition of the absence of disease, if the physician desires to confirm this condition or reduce the differential diagnosis, a highly specific examination will be of assistance. The question posed by the physician can be stated as, "If a patient does not have disease X, what is the likelihood of test Y being negative?"

The sensitivity and specificity of an exam have traditionally been a means of evaluating the capability of a testing system. In applying these probabilities to the diagnostic workup of a patient (pre-test phase of diagnosis), sensitivity and specificity should be used to recommend an appropriate exam.

The quality characteristics of sensitivity and specificity can provide a focus for improvement. For example, sensitivity and specificity are functions of the imaging devices (Are they calibrated? Do they meet today's imaging standards? Is quality control done regularly and correctly?), the exam being appropriately conducted, and the observational and interpretive skills of the reader, as well as the reading environment (recall the cause-and-effect diagram). All of these may be considered process variables that influence the quality characteristics of sensitivity and specificity.

A detailed examination of these areas may reveal room for improvement.

Evaluation of the Post-Test Product (Medical Decision Making)

The topic of scientific diagnostic decision making has evoked some strong reactions from practitioners of the "art" of medicine. Indeed, there is an art to the practice of medicine, and we should never lose sight of the attributes of caring and compassion required in the healthcare profession. Obviously, there is also a great deal of science in the practice of medicine. This section will peel away the myth that clinical diagnosis is strictly the art of intuitive thinking. There really is some scientific merit to the way that medicine is taught and practiced and how medical decisions are made.

After obtaining the results of the exam (i.e., post-test phase), the post-test likelihood that the patient does or does not have the disease, given that the test is positive or negative, is evaluated. If there is great certainty in the diagnosis, treatment of the patient may begin. If uncertainty remains, the testing phase must be revisited and it must be determined which exam will best serve the needs of the patient at this point in the diagnostic workup.

The measurable values in assessing post-test exam capability are as follows:

- **Positive predictive value (PPV):** TP/(TP + FP). The likelihood that a patient with a positive test has the disease.
- **Negative predictive value (NPV):** TN/(TN + FN). The likelihood that a patient with a negative test does not have the disease.
- **Post-test false-positive rate:** FP/(TP + FP) (1 − PPV). The likelihood that a patient with a positive test does not have the disease.
- **Post-test false-negative rate:** FN/(TN + FN) (1 − NPV). The likelihood that a patient with a negative test has the disease.

Once again, these definitions are examples of probabilities that have pre-conditions, i.e., conditional probabilities. After the exam, the following question is asked: "For a positive or negative test Y, what is the likelihood of the patient having disease X?" The post-test condition is that of a positive or negative test, and the probability or predictive value is the likelihood of the patient having or not having the disease given the condition of a positive or negative test. Note the reverse logic from the pre-test evaluation.

These are the values that are of the most use to a physician in deciding to treat the patient. The probabilities derived from this analysis are related to the diagnostic certainty.

There is a range of diagnostic certainty within which an immense amount of clinical knowledge and judgment play a significant role in decision making. Many physicians intuitively weigh the risk of treatment versus diagnostic certainty as well as the risk of continued testing in order to improve diagnostic certainty. While this model makes no attempt to address this intuitive process, it does help clarify the decision-making process which is necessary if quality improvement is to take place.

Improvement of Quality in Diagnostic Tests

A starting point in the quality improvement journey is to identify an ideal situation and measure how closely a test in the standard practice setting approximates its best known capability. K. N. Lohr defines efficacy and effectiveness as follows:

Efficacy: The level of benefit expected when health care services are applied under "ideal" conditions of use; hence, it refers to results that a technology could produce when applied by the most skilled practitioners in the best possible circumstances....

Effectiveness: The level of benefit when services are rendered under ordinary circumstances by average practitioners for typical patients.

Based on these definitions, when diagnostic tests in the standard practice setting are measured, they would have an effectiveness that could approach test efficacy. Assuming that effectiveness will be less than efficacy, any difference between the two can be measured as an opportunity for improvement. This sounds suspiciously similar to QA. The difference, however, is that systems and process, in addition to providers, are examined for potential improvement. In fact, it is anticipated that 85 to 90% of the problems associated with the difference between efficacy and effectiveness are the result of problems that exist in the system. TQM takes QA a step further in allowing for continued improvement once effectiveness reaches efficacy.

The quantitative measures of effectiveness and efficacy can include the characteristics of diagnostic tests described earlier: sensitivity, specificity, and positive and negative predictive values. These characteristics of test quality can be measured for any test for which an adequate "gold" standard can be defined.

Given a measure of quality, the improvement of that characteristic must come from a change in some aspect of the process by which that

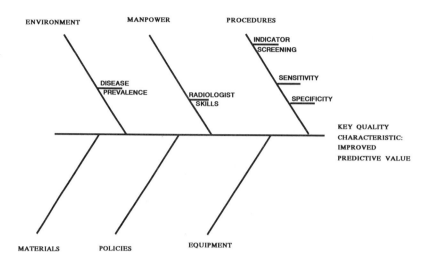

Figure 6.6 Cause-and-Effect Diagram for the Key Quality Characteristics of Predictive Values

quality is provided. Which aspect to change is determined by carefully evaluating those factors that influence the quality of the exam. This evaluation is carried out utilizing the tools of diagnostic improvement.

Once again, let's return to the cause-and-effect analysis for the key quality characteristic of predictive values. The variables that influence predictive values include the following key variables in the diagnostic process (Figure 6.6):

- Indications for the exam
- Sensitivity
- Specificity
- Diagnostic criteria
- Disease prevalence
- Knowledge of history, patient exam, and other exam results

We know from experience that there is a positive relationship between the predictive values of a positive examination and disease prevalence and a negative relationship with negative predictive values (Figures 6.7A and B). By pre-selecting patients for an exam (screening by histories and physician findings indicative of disease), the positive predictive values can be improved, and the cost of care can potentially be decreased by reducing the number of unnecessary exams.

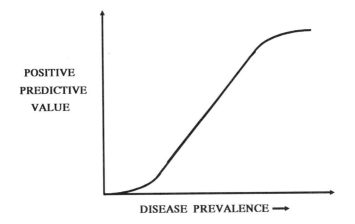

Figure 6.7A Positive Predictive Value vs. Disease Prevalence

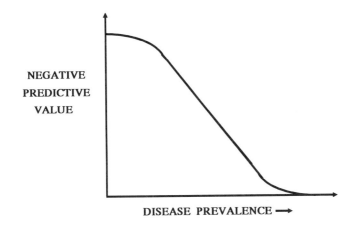

Figure 6.7B Negative Predictive Value vs. Disease Prevalence

SUMMARY

As illustrated in the above examples, improvement can be made anywhere in the diagnostic process. The challenge to healthcare professionals is to identify improvement scientifically and logistically where it will be of most benefit to the patient. If met, this challenge will also benefit the healthcare industry.

Part II

IMPLEMENTATION: MAKING IMPROVEMENT CONTINUOUS

7

The PROCESS
of GETTING STARTED

If there is no leadership from the top, stop promoting TQC.

Kaoru Ishikawa
What Is Total Quality Control

MAKING THE TRANSITION FROM BUSINESS AS USUAL

All successful managers are aware of the maxim that machines and inventory can be managed, but people must be led. The successful manager must be a leader of people. In undertaking a management change the magnitude of Total Quality Management (TQM), the leaders of the department must be knowledgeable in TQM and truly committed to its success.

Rule #1

The improvement effort must be driven by top management. This rule is so important that all other rules could be considered guidelines in comparison. Not only must the program have the blessing of top management, but it must also receive the support and resources necessary for its success. Top management must be actively involved. Personnel at all levels can see through empty promises. The cooperation needed will not materialize if top management does not demonstrate its full commitment.

A caveat is that it will take months to realize some of the first results and years to realize full implementation. In choosing this path, be prepared to stay the course and maintain focus on improvement and customer satisfaction.

The initial team should be composed of department leaders to establish an implementation plan and to serve as the driving force behind the quality improvement effort. Although the exact structure of the team may vary based on the size of the organization, a two-tiered organizational structure will serve most radiology departments well: a Quality Management Team (QMT) which guides the Quality Improvement Teams (QITs).

The QMT is a permanent team made up of the leadership (chairman, director/manager, quality improvement coordinator, chief technologists, etc.) of the radiology department. It may also include hospital quality improvement personnel. Its roles and functions are as follows:

1. Develop the vision, mission, and guiding principles for the radiology department (see Chapter 2).
2. Identify and remove any impediments to quality improvement (see Chapter 1).
3. Encourage employee participation in the QITs. An effective method is to hold a meeting with all department employees to explain the concept and objectives of these problem-solving teams.
4. Provide basic education on TQM for employees (see Chapter 3).
5. Select a project, a team leader, and a quality advisor who is knowledgeable in TQM.
6. Select a team.
7. Provide the necessary personnel, space, and other resources for the operation of the QITs.
8. Provide guidance and direction to the QITs.
9. Provide the QITs with the authority to implement solutions to problems, when feasible and practical.
10. Maintain open communication between the QMT and QITs.
11. Represent the interests of the team to the rest of the organization.

THE FUNDAMENTALS

Step #1: Vision, Mission, Guiding Principles

The first step in implementation is to review, rework, or draft a mission statement for the department. The vision statement and guiding principles should also become an integral part of the improvement process. Without them, the purpose is not as clear and goals may not be worthy of the time and resources dedicated to the improvement effort.

Step #2: Establish a TQM Knowledge Base

The second step in implementation is to improve the level of knowledge in the department about the quality improvement process. What is total quality management/total quality improvement? What tools are used? How are these tools applied? The fundamentals discussed in Chapters 1 to 5 serve the implementation process well. It is recommended that the history of TQM and Deming's 14 points be reviewed as a background for those unfamiliar with TQM. An overview of the tools of TQM is helpful, but further training in more detail will be needed when the improvement team begins its work.

Some facilities have conducted steps 1 and 2 simultaneously, and some have completed step 2 before step 1. The order at this point is not as critical as completing both before proceeding to step 3. Steps 1 and 2 only need to be accomplished once and will apply to all improvement projects. However, the vision and mission statements may require revision as time passes, as the medical environment changes, or as the vision, mission, and guiding principles are clarified through the improvement process.

Who Will Lead and Who Will Follow

Management literature is full of examples of implementing change. One lesson which has been learned is how personnel react to change. A change in management philosophy such as accompanies the implementation of TQM will encounter a similar response.

As illustrated in Figure 7.1, approximately 10% of the people will be ready for the change and embrace it (the pacesetters). The current and future leaders will probably be found within this group. On the other hand, another 10% will steadfastly be opposed to anything having to do with change (laggards). These people will probably have something to lose in the change. What they stand to lose may or may not be obvious. One manager, whose management style was to somewhat rule by fear and intimidation, professed a desire to implement TQM. However, resistance surfaced when it became apparent that the manager would have to give up this management style.

The remaining 80% will likely adopt a "wait and see" attitude before signing on. These are the people who will need to be shown how TQM can benefit them as well as the organization (a win–win situation). At this point they will know enough about TQM to maintain an open mind, but not enough to be able to put it into practice.

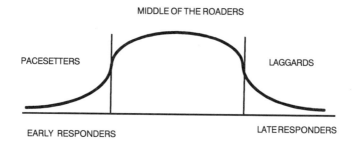

Figure 7.1 Personnel Response to Change

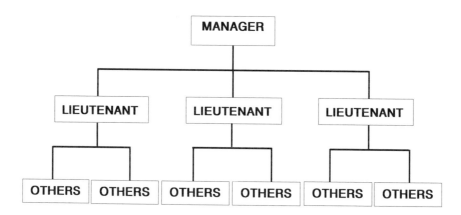

Figure 7.2 Traditional Structure

A word should also be said regarding the relationships encountered in the radiology department. Many departments have position or pyramid charts (Figure 7.2) that demonstrate who works for whom and who has what title, with the "most important" person on top and everyone else somewhere below. While responsibility and accountability are important to the structure of any organization, the concept that any one group or person is the most important is in need of revision. The team concept is illustrated in Figure 7.3, where all people fulfilling their responsibilities in relationship to the other groups is important to the overall function of the department. The loss of any one group is significantly detrimental to the operation and quality improvement.

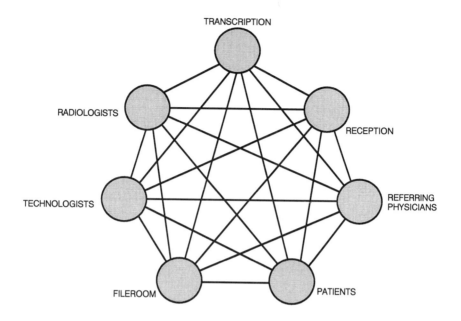

Figure 7.3 Departmental Relationships

Step #3: Find a Project (*F* of FOCUS-PDCA)

The third step is to determine the project(s) toward which the first efforts will be directed (Table 7.1). Early in the improvement process, those individuals with initiative and drive will want to solve all the problems at once. This is not recommended when implementing a management change the magnitude of TQM. Resources will be spread too thin and the likelihood of failure increased. The following are some guidelines to be used in establishing an improvement team:

1. Hospital and department leaders must be the first to learn and apply the quality improvement principles. Most leaders will find it difficult to lead others in something about which they know little or nothing.
2. Establish an organizational philosophy regarding team meetings. If overtime is necessary to accomplish the meetings, management must commit to the additional expense. It also may be helpful to encourage frequent meetings in the beginning, until the teams operate on their own.

Table 7.1 Project Selection Criteria

1.	Project well accepted
2.	Organizational benefit
3.	Relatively simple
4.	Rapid cycle time
5.	Well-defined beginning and end
6.	Serves the customers

3. Establish team membership with volunteers. It is helpful to begin with a sense of volunteerism on the part of those willing to study and apply continuous improvement in their work areas. Peer pressure will soon bring others into the process.

4. Train the members in the basics of quality improvement. In order to succeed, workers must have the appropriate tools. Problem solving, basic statistics, and data collection and evaluation are essential to continuous problem solving.

5. Establish the continuous improvement function of the improvement team. Ensure that the team members understand that their purpose is continuous improvement, rather than just solving one specific problem. The essential points for which they are responsible should be continuously examined for ways to improve them.

6. Department leaders must regularly attend and participate in team meetings. The extent of their interest will determine the success of the teams. This is essential not only to show support for the total quality improvement efforts, but also to maintain stability and leadership in the transition. At times, the newfound empowerment can result in liberties which may result in costly setbacks if not carefully thought through and approved by a top-down-driven QMT.

7. The QIT is the foundation of total quality improvement. While the TQM philosophy is based on support from the top of the organization, the true expertise and capacity for improvement comes from those closest to the problems.

Step #4: Organize the Quality Improvement Team (O of FOCUS-PDCA)

Implementing TQM is a process in and of itself, and the organization is best served by careful step-by-step planning and by educating personnel in the transformation. In organizations in which there is great enthusiasm for change, large numbers of people have been successfully educated in the methods and philosophies of TQM, whereas in organizations where there is greater resistance to change, small projects may be necessary to demonstrate its value.

In either case, it is critical to the success of the implementation to choose a project that:

1. Will be well accepted by all who influence the process
2. Will be beneficial for the organization
3. Is relatively simple
4. Has a rapid cycle time (i.e., information can be easily obtained and analyzed, so that the effects of changes made can be quickly realized)
5. Has a process with a well-defined beginning and end
6. Serves the needs and expectations of the external customers

In actually making the selection, in some organizations upper management has selected the process to be improved. The preferred method, however, is to let the people who will be doing the improving select what they are to improve, provided that they are given guidelines similar to those in the previous paragraph and provided that customer satisfaction/complaints suggest the need for change. This serves several purposes: (1) it reinforces empowerment, (2) it fosters the involvement of those people who most likely know what is wrong, and (3) it engenders the respect and trust which management must have for all the personnel.

In one situation, the people involved in departmental improvement selected patient waiting time as the number one process to be improved. They did so because (1) it was well accepted by all who influenced or contributed to patient waiting time, (2) it benefited the organization (improved patient and referring physician satisfaction and increased patient volume/revenues), (3) it was relatively simple to measure and had a rapid cycle time (waiting times could be monitored daily and the effects of changes could be seen), (4) it had a well-defined process beginning (patient arrives) and end (patient departs), and (5) it served the needs and expectations of the external customers (patients provided direct feedback in that they either were complimentary about the brief waiting time or complained about the excess delay). Management only heard complaints about delays that were well beyond reason, which were few.

Once the process for improvement has been selected, it is as critical to choose the members of the improvement team as it was to select the process. The team that sees its purpose as solving problems with quality and effectiveness is the backbone of the improvement effort.

MANAGING THE IMPLEMENTATION

Broad-based involvement by all levels of employees, along with the total commitment of top management, is essential to implementing continuous quality improvement. The necessity of and requirements for the QMT were previously discussed. With the project selected, focus moves to the team that will be studying and improving the process: the QIT (Table 7.2).

The QIT is a small group of employees who meet at regular intervals to identify, analyze, and solve problems related to quality, productivity, cost, and safety. Members of the team are volunteers who have a stake in the process to be improved. The volunteers must be committed to participating in the process of improvement. However, to ensure success, other workers with an intimate knowledge of the process to be improved should be invited to join the team. The success of the team will be determined by the extent of the commitment to participate.

In identifying the key workers to be invited, the following questions need to be answered:

- What is the process to be improved?
- Who is close to the problem?
- Who is accountable for ("owns") the process?
- Who has the expertise?
- Who should be consulted?

Roles and Functions of Quality Improvement Team Members

Leader

Initially, a radiology supervisor or manager may be the most suitable team leader. Once the quality team has become functional and members are familiar with the process, it is best to have the team elect its own leader.

The leader is the manager of the team. He or she makes arrangements for meetings, sets agendas, oversees preparation of reports, and orchestrates the activities of the team. The leader should be good at working with individuals and groups. The scope of his or her responsibilities includes:

- The point of contact between the team and the QMT.
- The keeper of the team's records and data.
- If the leader is a supervisor, he or she retains the authority vested in that position. Therefore, changes within the area of authority of the supervisor can be immediately implemented following approval by the team.

Table 7.2 QIT Membership

Leader	Owner of the process
Recorder	Keeper of the records
Timekeeper	Moves the meeting along
Members	Active participants in the improvement process
Facilitator	Quality improvement specialist and team resource

Recorder

A single designated member of the team should be responsible for keeping the written record of activities that take place at each meeting. Although at first glance this may appear to be unnecessary paperwork, the importance of record keeping cannot be overemphasized in view of the continuous nature of the activity of the team and the large number of ideas generated. The recorded minutes are also extremely helpful in evaluation of the team by the QMT.

The recorder should be able to take notes rapidly and accurately. He or she should be willing to speak out to request that participants speak one at a time or more slowly.

The recorded minutes should include the following information:

- Name of the team
- Date and time of the meeting
- Names of those present and absent
- Action taken to review and approve the minutes of the previous meeting
- Each agenda item deliberated
  - Major points, questions, problems, or concerns
  - Every suggestion generated by brainstorming
  - Agreements, decisions, or actions
- Presentations
- Assignments or follow-up activities with due dates or deadlines
- Tentative agenda of the next meeting
- Date and time of the next meeting
- Time of adjournment

Timekeeper

The timekeeper helps the team manage its time. The timekeeper calls out the time remaining for each item on the agenda at intervals determined by team. It is the team's responsibility to manage time, and the timekeeper simply assists the team in this process.

Members

The QIT is made up of approximately five to ten members. Members are selected because they work in, own, supply, or benefit from the process that is the focus of the team.

Team members collect data and continually study the process they are trying to improve. During meetings, members share information and data and participate in making decisions and developing plans.

Facilitator

The facilitator has special expertise in the quality improvement process. He or she is not actually a member of the team, but rather serves as a coach or consultant to the team. The facilitator helps the QIT get started and works with the team in collecting and interpreting data and developing plans to improve the process that is being studied. The facilitator *does not* set the agenda, obtain information related to the subject matter, or make decisions. The role of the facilitator decreases as the QIT acquires more experience.

The Meeting Process

Planning

The team leader and facilitator need to set guidelines as the first order of business. These guidelines should identify:

- The primary objective of the team
- How often meetings will be held
- The extent of training to be provided to the team members
- How the effectiveness of the team will be evaluated

Set an Agenda

Meetings are typically one hour in length. In early meetings, ten minutes is devoted to reviewing any open items remaining from the last meeting. Twenty minutes is used for new training material, and the remaining half hour is assigned to discussion of the team project.

The following agenda is recommended for the very first meeting of the team:

1. Self introduction by team members (10 minutes)
2. Discuss the purpose of the team (20 minutes)
3. Define roles of the team leader, facilitator, recorder, timekeeper, and members (10 minutes)

4. Review FOCUS-PDCA and establish a "road map" or time line of goals for the team (40 minutes)
5. Assignments for the next meeting (5 minutes)

Set a Site, Environment, and Time

Although seemingly unimportant, the location and environment of the meeting site can often mean the difference between success and failure. A meeting conducted in the Board room may not yield better results, but, on the other hand, a crowded, dirty, noisy room is definitely not conducive to discussion of quality. A clean, uncluttered room with adequate seating and adequate space for flip charts or a chalk board is a minimum requirement.

Team meetings should be scheduled regularly (usually once a week). Meetings typically last one hour and should ideally be held during working hours. If members attend team meetings on overtime, they should be paid overtime wages. However, holding meetings during normal working hours is strongly recommended because it drives home the point that quality is a routine part of the business day, rather than an afterthought or additional responsibility.

Work the Agenda

A written detailed agenda distributed at least a day before the meeting is a prerequisite for an effective meeting. This allows team members to come to the meeting prepared and alleviates common causes of confusion at the beginning of the meeting.

Apart from the content of the meeting, starting and ending the meeting on time is important in making the meeting productive. The leader should adhere to the following guidelines in order to effectively manage a meeting:

1. Encourage group members to speak up. Draw out the more reticent members by asking for their opinions and ideas.
2. Balance the discussion; maintain a non-partisan, non-judgmental position.
3. Keep the discussion on track. Do not let members digress; redirect the discussion back to the issues at hand.
4. Avoid controversial issues at the beginning of the meeting.
5. Finish on schedule.

To handle an overly talkative team member, ask him or her to summarize the major points of the discussion and then invite reaction from other members. Discourage side conversation by asking the member to share the discussion with the entire team. The team leader should hold back his or her opinion until other team members have had a chance to be heard.

To get through the agenda, stick to the allotted time for each topic. End the meeting by reaching a conclusion and initiating positive action.

Assign Follow-Up Activities

A well-planned and well-run meeting will be worthless unless the words are turned into actions. The team leader should assign team members to the specific activities approved by the team and reach agreement on when the tasks should be accomplished. Assistance should be provided as needed.

One or two days after the meeting, the team leader should send out minutes of the meeting. The minutes should include the pending actions, persons responsible, and anticipated schedule of completion. The leader should also check with those members assigned a task to determine their progress or identify barriers that threaten failure. Assistance should be provided as needed.

Evaluate the Meeting

The last act in each meeting should be an evaluation of the team process. The following questions should be answered by all team members and evaluated by the leader and facilitator:

1. Was time used effectively during the meeting?
2. Were all team members prepared?
3. Were individual assignments completed?
4. What were the weaknesses of today's meeting?
5. What went well that we should continue doing?
6. How can we improve the next meeting?

PITFALLS

Process Selection Problems

Choosing a system rather than a process: Selecting an ambitious project that transcends departmental boundaries or has a large number of inputs and variables may lead to frustration because of the complexity of the problems encountered. A system can be defined as consisting of numerous processes and having numerous owners, suppliers, and missions. In the beginning, if faced with a system in disarray (such as purchasing supplies) where other departments influence the process, it is preferable to select a segment of purchasing that is under the control of the department and improve this part of the process first. Make sure your own house is in order before trying to support improvements in other external departments.

Choosing a process undergoing change from another source: An example of this would be studying the process of manually maintaining patient files while another source is designing the implementation of a computerized radiology information system. This wastes the time of those studying the manual information system because it will become obsolete with the installation of the computerized system. An appropriate action would be to combine the two groups and pool expertise and resources in order to integrate the results.

Choosing a solution rather than a process: Leaders pushing the implementation of TQM can occasionally confuse the process with the desirable outcome. This undermines the sense of empowerment promoted by continuous quality improvement. More importantly, it undermines the tenet of effectively delegating responsibility, which is part of any good management program. Review the sample opportunity statements. The statement should not suggest a solution, but instead should allow a solution to be developed by studying the process.

Choosing a "pet" project of little interest to others: Another pitfall is selecting a project of limited interest or of interest only to management. This should be done with great caution. It should be done only if it will be possible to convince those involved in the improvement process that it is important to address the issue at this time. Studying processes and analyzing data is at times difficult work. At those times, the only motivation to continue may be the hope of future improvement and a more desirable workplace. "Pet" projects that fail to obtain the commitment of the workers will suffer from inattention.

Team Selection

If organizing a QIT is expected to be a "quick fix," it is sure to fail. In the absence of department-wide implementation of TQM, QITs will not be productive for long.

Voluntary participation of departmental employees in the QIT is key to success. Selected employees, however, may be invited to participate in the initial team. Any real or perceived coercion to participate in the team activity will be counterproductive.

Sometimes there may be more volunteers than the ideal size of the team can accommodate. Instead of accepting all interested individuals and ending up with an unmanageable team, it is advisable for the team leader to select a manageable number of team members (four to six) and counsel the remaining volunteers that there will be other opportunities in the near future and quality people will be needed to participate in those teams. This works only when an atmosphere of mutual trust and respect exists between workers and management, built on many years of promises that are made and kept.

Process Ownership

An important premise of TQM is that the workers closest to the problem are more likely to know what is wrong with a process and how to fix it, because of their intimate knowledge of job conditions.

Refer to Chapter 4 for a review of how to identify the owner of a process in the radiology department. If the owner of the process to be improved is not a regular member of the team, he or she should be included as an ad hoc member.

Lack of a Game Plan

The best laid schemes o'mice and men
Gang aft a – gley:
An' Lea'e us naught but grief and pain,
for promis'd joy.

Robert Burns

The only way to avoid frustration is to have a clear concept of what is to be accomplished. The primary objective of the team, whether personal and team development, measurable gains, or some combination of both, must be clearly stated, along with the permissible scope of the quality or productivity improvement.

A workable game plan should combine the following requirements:

1. List of all specific activities to be completed
2. Sequence of activities from start to completion
3. Identification of time required to complete each activity
4. Who will complete each activity

Staying the Course

It will take years to fully implement a program such as TQM. In the beginning, many employees may be skeptical of the QIT concept. They may equate this process with other failed quality projects imposed by management. However, if the department managers remain enthusiastically committed to the principles of TQM, the cumulative yield over time will be gratifying.

The initiation of project teams will produce a variety of emotions. The initial enthusiasm for the newfound empowerment and commitment will likely turn to discouragement and frustration when the real work begins. The people participating have not yet developed the skill and experience necessary to consistently use the tools of TQM. The cost of implementing quality will likely increase during this time. It is essential that all involved stay focused on the vision and mission. This will quickly result in exhilaration when the first improvements are realized or the first milestones are successfully reached.

In time, as the team continues to pursue continuous quality improvement, its members will become much more knowledgeable about applying the tools of TQM and settle into a feeling of control over the process for which they are responsible. They will feel a sense of satisfaction in realizing that it is their efforts that have contributed to the success. It is important to share this expected passage with the team as they experience it and encourage them to continue their efforts.

Resistance to Change

Supervisors are key to the successful implementation of TQM in a radiology department. This group is often better educated, more knowledgeable, and accustomed to problem solving. They may also, however, be the most resistant to change, because they are required to practice a participative decision-making process with the employees they supervise.

Lack of Team Building

Failure to weld the team into a group committed to a common purpose will result in inefficiency or failure. It is important that the facilitator and team leader understand team dynamics and know how to react to team problems. (An excellent source of information is *The Team Handbook* by Peter Scholtes (Joiner Associates, Madison, Wisc.)

Failure to Educate the Team

People cannot be expected to succeed if they are not given the tools necessary to get the job done. When the improvement teams are expected to find and fix problems without being provided the wherewithal to do the job, they most certainly will fail. The most important responsibility of the facilitator is to ensure that the team receives appropriate training as needed. The most important responsibility of management is to ensure that these training resources are available.

8

IMPROVEMENT in DEPARTMENT LOGISTICS

The individual components of the system, instead of being competitive, will for optimization reinforce each other for accomplishment of the aim of the system.

W. Edwards Deming
The New Economics

As stated in Chapter 3, areas for improvement have been divided into logistics (assisting patients through the exam process, supplying the needs of the department, completing the final product, etc.) and diagnostic science (the scientific assessment of the diagnostic and therapeutic product). Each has its own particular methods and processes, and TQM can be applied to each in an effort to continually improve the product.

The examples discussed in this chapter are universal in that they probably have been encountered at most facilities and are easily understood. The treatment here is meant to be instructive rather than an exhaustive evaluation of the topic.

Because facilities studied herein are in the early phase of implementing TQM, no final solutions or long-term assessments can be made from these examples. The examples should provide the reader with a good idea of how he or she might address these and other problems from a TQM approach and graphically illustrate how the tools of TQM can be applied. While some of the solutions may seem trivial and the graphs and data unnecessary, bear in mind that this presentation is intended to be instructive. Remaining true to the principles of TQM in the simple early projects increases the likelihood of success in dealing with the more complicated problems that will be faced in the future.

This chapter begins with a discussion of the importance of clarifying the mission of the department. Four case studies of TQM problem solving are then provided, based on actual experiences in radiology departments. The four examples are patient waiting time, report turnaround time, patient access, and missed revenues. These examples are intended to assist the reader in further understanding the TQM approach to continuous quality improvement.

CLARIFYING THE MISSION OF THE DEPARTMENT

As discussed in Chapter 2, everyone involved in quality improvement must have a clear idea of the mission of the organization in order to contribute fully and effectively.

One facility took it upon itself to define a vision, mission, and guiding principles before undertaking quality improvement. This is the recommended approach. Others have done little more than ensure that the team has clear goals and purpose. Teams that have neither clear goals nor purpose have uniformly failed to achieve anything but wasted time and perhaps an appreciation of the need for goals and purpose.

Chapter 2 should be reviewed before initiating any quality improvement project. In addition, all who volunteer to participate in the improvement process should also be allowed to participate in developing a statement of purpose for the team and establishing goals which support that purpose.

TACKLING EXCESSIVE PATIENT WAITING TIME

In evaluating patient complaints, a large medical center with a sizable outpatient clinic found that the most frequent complaint on patient satisfaction surveys was excessive waiting time. As a result, patients would find other facilities from which to obtain their outpatient diagnostic imaging or would leave dissatisfied with the service rendered.

One of the most important facets of medical practice is gaining and maintaining the confidence of the patient. This is not appreciably different in many other industries. One major airline reminds their cabin service personnel that the cleanliness of the seats and trays translates into confidence in the airline. From the passenger's perspective, if the cabin is a mess, is engine maintenance likely to be much better?

The timeliness of the exam and the courtesy with which the patient is treated directly translate into the quality of care as perceived by the patient. Most patients are unfamiliar with such factors as film quality and skill of the interpreter. Therefore, the best film technique and the most astute diagnosis will be meaningless to the patient facing long waiting times and discourteous treatment.

Recognizing this, at one facility the department leadership and interested members with background training in TQM reviewed their vision and mission statements. It was obvious that excessive waiting times satisfied neither the statements of service nor the patients. Patient waiting time was selected as the process most likely to have the greatest impact on patient satisfaction. In the parlance of FOCUS-PDCA (see Chapter 4), they **F**ound their problem.

In defining the problem, the beginning and end points must be identified and the boundaries within which the improvement process will take place must be established. This department chose to limit their study to walk-in outpatient waiting times. The beginning of the process was identified as the time the patient presented at the reception desk and the end was the time the patient was released from the department.

They defined the current situation and identified what was wrong with it and why it needed improvement. A desirable result of the improvement process was also defined. Their opportunity statement read as follows:

> An opportunity to improve patient waiting time exists in the XYZ Radiology Department, beginning with the time the patient arrives in the department and ending with the time the patient is dismissed. The current examination process creates excessive waiting times and patient and physician dissatisfaction in that patients spend time with nothing to do and the referring physician's clinic is delayed waiting for results in order to make therapeutic decisions. Receptionists and technologists are made less efficient because of the time it takes to respond to the many patients who want to know how much longer their wait will be. The radiologist is dissatisfied by the time expended and the many interruptions to ask whether he or she has the films for the inquiring patient. Improvement should result in decreased patient waiting times, improved patient and physician satisfaction, and improved receptionist, technologist, and radiologist efficiency and satisfaction.

Let's take this statement apart.

> An opportunity to improve patient waiting time exists in the XYZ Radiology Department, beginning with the time the patient arrives in the department and ending with the time the patient is dismissed.

This defines the focus of the improvement effort (waiting time) and the boundaries (arrival through dismissal).

> The current examination process creates excessive waiting times and patient and physician dissatisfaction in that patients spend time with nothing to do and the referring physician's clinic is delayed waiting for results in order to make therapeutic decisions. Receptionists and technologists are made less efficient because of the time it takes to respond to the many patients who want to know how much longer their wait will be. The radiologist is dissatisfied by the time expended and the many interruptions to ask whether he or she has the films for the inquiring patient.

This defines the problem and its related issues in specific and measurable terms (time) and the impact of performance (efficiency). It should be obvious why it is important that this problem be solved.

> Improvement should result in decreased patient waiting times, improved patient and physician satisfaction, and improved receptionist, technologist, and radiologist efficiency and satisfaction.

This describes who or what will benefit (patients, referring physicians, radiologists, technologists, and receptionists), specifies a result (decreased waiting time), and does not imply any root causes or solutions. It also does not fix blame.

It is important to note that the result in this opportunity statement (decreased waiting time) is specific but allows for continuous improvement. Recall that the purpose of the team is to reduce patient waiting time. An initial goal may be a waiting time of less than 30 minutes, but the purpose of the team is still to reduce waiting time. Therefore, a goal of 25 minutes may become the new standard to be achieved.

An analogy of travel is appropriate in discussing purpose. If the purpose is to travel west, that purpose is satisfied by traveling from New York to Chicago, then to Denver, San Francisco, Honolulu, Hong Kong, New Delhi, and Paris. Each stop represents a goal achieved, and each satisfies the purpose of traveling west. In patient waiting time, the purpose is to reduce the wait. Any statistically significant improvement can be considered a goal achieved.

Management wanted a baseline sample of waiting time to establish a benchmark in order to determine whether any improvement resulted from the efforts of the team. A simple form was drafted and the outpatient population seeking exams was sampled for a one-week period as a pilot study. An average waiting time was determined from this sample.

The next task was to select a team (**O**rganize a team) to continue definition and improvement of the process. Volunteers were solicited, and some individuals were invited to participate. Leaders in the areas that contributed to producing the exams were asked to participate in and support the improvement project. Representatives were included from reception, technologists working in the outpatient area of the radiology department, the file room, and radiologists assigned to the "wet reading" desk.

When the team first met, the person most likely to be responsible for patient throughput was elected team leader. In this example, the chief technologist was elected. A timekeeper and a recorder were also selected. Training was initiated to identify the responsibilities of each member and the purpose of the team. The opportunity statement was reviewed and no modifications were necessary. It was established that the team would meet weekly for 1 hour during normal working hours. The next meeting would focus on the process of serving patients needing radiographic examinations.

C (Clarify the Problem): Specifying Current Patient Flow

Following training in flowcharting, the process of a fictional average patient passing through the department to obtain a radiograph was charted. Team members frequently recognized that current procedures were not very efficient when viewing the entire process. Numerous attempts to redefine the process were made during the meeting. The leader and facilitator stressed that the purpose of this step was to identify the *current* process. The finished product is presented in Figure 8.1.

Obvious Improvements

Team members quickly recognized areas for improvement but agreed to make changes only when they could be classified as obvious improvements (all members agreed that the improvement was obvious, would have no adverse effect on another process, would not change the activities of customers or suppliers). This was an eye-opening exercise. Members frequently mentioned how confusing and insensitive some of the processes were for patients and each other.

As an example, the file room noted that its policy was to collect pull notices until five or six were accumulated; the film jackets for the batch were then sent to the quality control area to be matched with the films. This created a delay of up to 45 minutes in some cases. Recognizing that this routine contributed to patient delay, the file room began pulling film jackets upon receipt of a pull notice, which immediately reduced the

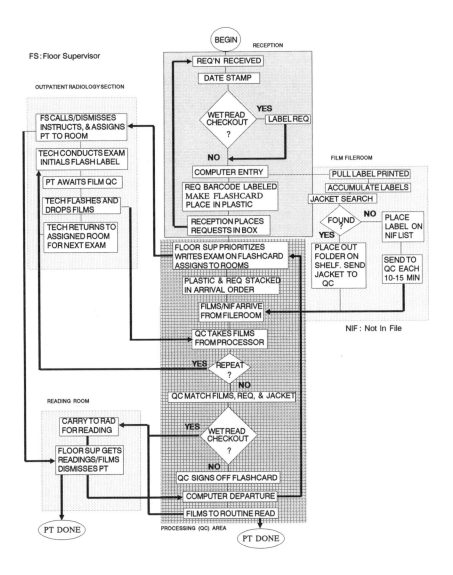

Figure 8.1 Patient Throughput Flowchart

pull time to less than 5 minutes—an obvious improvement. Figure 8.2, which is a section of the entire flowchart, indicates where in the flowchart this delay was found.

Other steps were found to be variable. People had differing ideas as to their responsibilities. In these cases, the process could not be charted as *current* because no consensus was reached. For example, when the

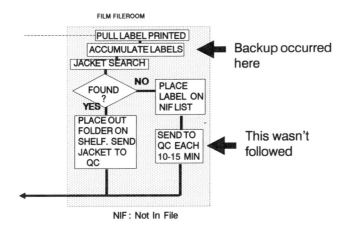

Figure 8.2 Patient Throughput Flowchart: File Room

flashcard was printed and transferred from the reception area to the technologist area, some receptionists placed the priority of the exam on the flashcard, some kept the cards in order of arrival, and in some cases the technologists could choose among the flashcards to select the exam they wanted to perform rather that picking the highest priority item or one that had been there for the longest period of time. The team leader, with the consensus of the team members, defined the new routine and then used PDCA to implement this obvious change.

In planning the implementation of this change, the team reviewed the steps of PDCA:

1. Set goals and define methods to reach them.
2. Engage in education and training.
3. Implement the work change.
4. Check the effects of the implementation.
5. Take appropriate action to sustain the gain or rethink the plan.

The goal remained to minimize patient waiting time. The method was defined by the team. Team and section leaders consulted to determine how personnel would be educated about the change, when the training would take place, and when the change would go into effect. This was accomplished and monitored by section leaders to ascertain whether the change was effective. In comparison to the patient waiting time database, there was an immediate improvement in the time patients waited for an X-ray room.

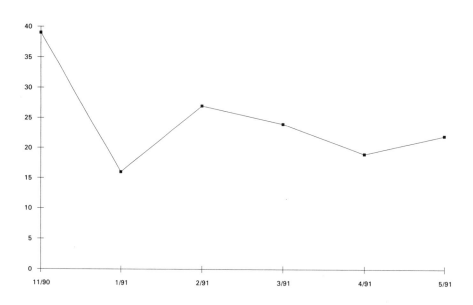

Figure 8.3 Time from Reception to Room

Figure 8.3 is a comparison of the situation before and after the change. When the benchmark sample was obtained in November 1990, the average time patients waited before entering an examination room once they had registered was nearly 40 minutes. After changing exam priorities and room assignments and defining responsibilities in the process, the immediate result was a decrease in waiting time to just over 15 minutes.

The observant reader will note that the next sample showed that the average wait increased to over 25 minutes. This will be further examined in the discussion of **A** (Act) of PDCA.

Data Collection

Obtaining usable data is essential in order for the team to proceed. The original time forms (disliked by the technologists and reception personnel) were now viewed as important improvement tools and in need of revision. Patient type was added, and several other time slots were added to further define areas that obstructed the flow. Planning for introduction of the next change occurred as it had with the procedural changes undertaken before.

Data Needed

Date of exam

Type of exam

Patient type (emergency room, urgent care, routine, etc.)

Arrival time

Time patient taken to X-ray room

Time exam quality controlled

Time patient dismissed

A time slip containing boxes for the above information was drafted. Approximately every fifth patient was evaluated by attaching the slip to the requisition that followed the patient through the department. A sample of this form is provided in Appendix A. When the team realized that something could be learned from those patients whose waiting times exceeded three standard deviations, the patient ID number was added to the time slip.

A database was developed to process and analyze the data collected. By properly filtering the database, a tremendous amount of information could be retrieved (Figure 8.4A). The database contained dates, times, and patient and exam types, which were used to stratify the data when assembled for analysis. The database fields (CHK-RM, time from reception to entering the exam room; RM-CMPLT, time from entering the room until the exam was judged complete; READ, time to match the study with the film jacket and interpret/dictate the exam; and T_WAIT, the total time the patient waited in the department) are calculated fields; that is, they are calculated by the database program by subtracting the time differentials from the times entered in the database. The error #VALUE! indicates that no reading time was entered and was used to identify those exams which were not "wet read."

This information not only yields average times for each interval, but can be stratified, or sorted, by patient type, time of day, and day of the week (Figure 8.4B). A spreadsheet display of the data is helpful in making decisions based on good information. For example, the average time a patient waits for an exam room, the average time to complete the exam, the average time to read the exam, and the average total wait are all computed for each patient type and exam type. In addition, average times are displayed for the time of day the patient arrived in order to assess waiting time as a function of time of day.

Maximum, minimum, and standard deviation are also calculated to facilitate constructing control and trend charts. The actual number of sampled patients in each of the sorts is also displayed to yield validation of the data. A sample of 3 would not have much credibility, but a sample of 100 would be considered representative of outpatient waiting time.

DATE	CHEST	OUTPT	ER	INPATIENT	URG	CHECKIN	ROOM	COMPLETE	READING	CHK-RM	RM-CMPLT	READ	T_WAIT
05/01/90	X				X	0940	0955	1006		15	11	#VALUE!	26
05/01/90	X				X	0904	0930	0938		26	8	#VALUE!	34
05/01/90			X		X	0930	0957	1002		27	5	#VALUE!	32
05/01/90		X				0904	0908	0921		4	13	#VALUE!	17
05/03/90		X			X	1025	1110	1125		45	15	#VALUE!	60
05/03/90		X			X	1202	1218	1234		16	16	#VALUE!	32
05/03/90	X		X			1100	1132	1220	1500	32	48	160	240
05/04/90	X				X	1317	1321	1329		4	8	#VALUE!	12
05/04/90	X		X			1305	1325	1333		20	8	#VALUE!	28
05/04/90		X	X			1200	1210	1221		10	11	#VALUE!	21
05/04/90					X	1136	1150	1155	1200	14	5	5	24
05/04/90					X	1145	1155	1159	1201	10	4	2	16
05/04/90					X	1115	1125	1130	1207	10	5	37	52
05/04/90			X			1121	1135	1141		14	6	#VALUE!	20
05/04/90		X	X		X	1012	1024	1040	1053	12	16	13	41
05/04/90						1017	1030	1040	1055	13	10	15	38
05/04/90					X	1016	1025	1040		9	15	#VALUE!	24
05/04/90	X				X	0950	1000	1024	1053	10	24	29	63
05/04/90	X				X	0928	0942	0954	1000	14	12	6	32
05/04/90	X				X	0901	0915	0935	0955	14	20	20	54

Figure 8.4A Waiting Time Database

	CKIN-RM	RM-CMPLT	READ	TOTAL	NUM PTS	3STDEV	MAX	MIN	NUM READS
WET READS	16.33	14.60	24.07	55.00	43	86	160.00	25.00	43
NON WETS	21.85	11.18	N/A	33.03	78	56	125.00	9.00	0
INPTS	18.09	9.73	N/A	27.82	11	48	60.00	9.00	0
ADINUNIF	17.33	11.97	11.75	32.43	30	71	137.00	10.00	8
ER PTS	11.00	13.00	19.43	43.43	7	44	76.00	33.00	7
OTHERS	22.05	12.92	28.75	46.00	73	78	160.00	15.00	28
CHEST	20.64	9.80	26.70	36.87	83	72	160.00	9.00	20
OTHER EX	18.38	17.48	21.67	48.24	42	73	137.00	20.00	24
OVERALL	19.88	12.40	24.07	40.83	121	75	160.00	9.00	43
0700-0800	16.00	24.67	5.00	42.33	3	58	55.00	20.00	1
0800-0900	12.50	11.71	40.57	44.50	14	111	160.00	9.00	7
0900-1000	19.54	10.20	20.91	36.31	35	63	105.00	10.00	11
1000-1100	24.45	13.45	21.29	45.74	38	81	137.00	15.00	14
1100-1200	15.67	11.33	31.40	40.08	12	67	82.00	15.00	5
1200-1300	17.86	15.14	12.50	36.57	7	74	88.00	15.00	2
1300-1400	12.00	11.67	8.00	26.33	3	7	29.00	25.00	1
1400-1500	29.83	14.33	9.00	45.67	6	58	76.00	23.00	1
1500-1600	18.50	10.50	19.00	38.50	2	6	40.00	37.00	1
MAX	29.83	24.67	40.57	55.00					
MIN	11.00	9.73	5.00	26.33					

% WET READS   35.54

Figure 8.4B Post-Processing of the Waiting Time Database

With the problem defined, the patient flow outlined, and obvious improvements made, the cause of the variation needs to be identified.

U (Understanding the Causes of Process Variation): Identifying Delays

The concept of customer and supplier was reinforced to the team once the flowchart was completed. Each part of the chart was divided into a basic process (supplier, input, action, output, customer) and each was defined. For example, in the process of communicating the need for an exam from the reception desk to the technologists, the reception personnel are the suppliers, the technologists are the internal customers (the patient is the external customer), the input is the exam and patient information, the action is production of a completed request and flashcard, and the output is a complete request and flashcard with priority assigned. A process worksheet similar to Figure 8.5 is usually helpful early in the implementation process to assist in keeping things clear.

Quality characteristics were identified and key quality characteristics chosen for each basic process. Variables that affected the key quality characteristics were identified and displayed graphically on a fishbone diagram (Figure 8.6). For example, one of the quality characteristics chosen by the radiologist (internal customer of the exam reading process) was the presence of a film jacket with comparison films for chest radiographs.

Only about 20% of the chest radiographs presented for interpretation had previous studies available for comparison. Researching the causes identified the information shown in Figure 8.7 (a Pareto chart). Clearly, the major reason no comparisons were available was because the film jacket had been checked out. In addition, most of the time it had been checked out by the clinic that was requesting a new film.

The long-standing policy of checking out film jackets on patients the evening before their appointments resulted in considerable rework on the part of the file room staff. They searched for and pulled the films the evening before the exam and sent the jackets to the clinics requesting them. When the patients presented the next day for radiographic examination, the file room, unaware that the films had already been checked out, conducted another search. They then found that the films had been checked out. However, the fact that they had been checked out was not communicated to the processing area, and the films were presented to the radiologist for reading with the notation "NIF" (not in file). The radiologist then indicated that comparison films must be found

PROCESS WORKSHEET						
Proc #	Supplier	input	Action	Output	Customer	Needs and Expectations
1	Recept	Pt Info	Complete request Computer entry Deliver to Techs	PPWK	Lead tech Patient	Accurate paperwork in a minimum of time from the pt arrival Courtesy, minimum wait, accurate information transmitted
2	Lead Tech	Priorities Avail Rm	Assigns room, exam	Flashcard w/ room, exam, & priority	Tech Patient	Accurate paperwork in a minimum of time from the pt arrival Courtesy, minimum wait, accurate information transmitted
3						
4						

Figure 8.5 Process Worksheet

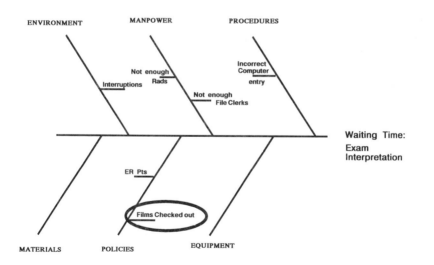

Figure 8.6 Cause-and-Effect Diagram

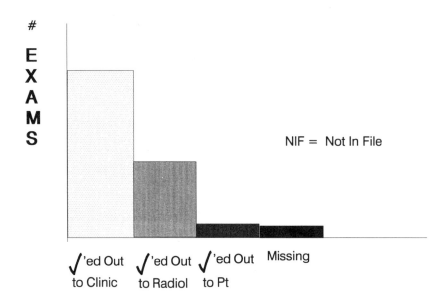

Figure 8.7 Causes of Films Not in File

in order to provide a reasonable interpretation, which resulted in another search to find the cause, which was that the jacket had been checked out to the clinic that requested the radiographic exam.

S (Selecting the Best Current Solution): Information-Based Decision Making

In attacking the greatest contributor to waiting time, it was hypothesized that by not checking out the film jackets prior to the patient's exam, the exam could be compared, the quality and significance of the interpretation would be improved, and the patient would not be delayed while the file room conducted an additional search. This problem was solved by asking the requesting clinics to check out the films after the exam rather than prior to sending the patient.

This solution fulfilled the requirement that the clinics have the films for the patient appointment and met the radiology department's need to reduce patient waiting time. It was an obvious win–win situation.

Little remained static as the improvement program progressed. In analyzing the waiting times for each segment of the process (from the spreadsheet display of monthly data), excess waits for readings also

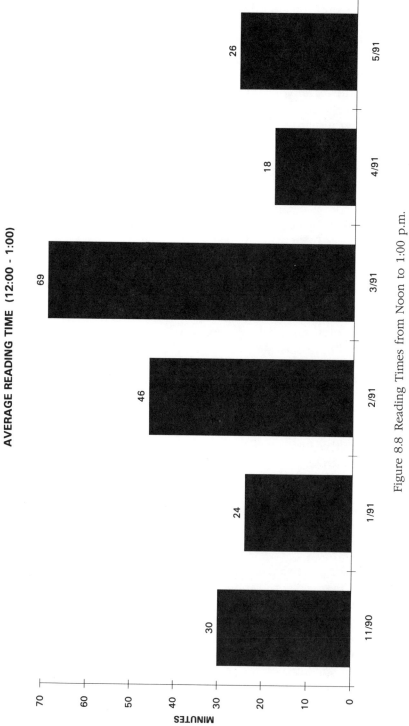

Figure 8.8 Reading Times from Noon to 1:00 p.m.

appeared around the noon hour in the fourth month (Figure 8.8). In identifying this special cause, it was determined that the radiologist charged with noon coverage was at the noon conference, which the technologists did not want to interrupt. As a result, the exams piled up until the radiologist returned to the current and backlogged "wet" reads. Instructing the technologists to notify the radiologists of "wet" readings solved this problem, and indeed a remarkable improvement occurred the following month.

Staffing was another area where information supported operational decisions. How many technologists were needed? By evaluating patient waiting times during differing staffing levels and patient loads, it was possible to identify an optimal staffing level. It is well known that systems do not necessarily work better simply by adding personnel. By plotting patient waiting time against technologists per exam load, the optimal staffing for the number of rooms available at the facility was determined. Figure 8.9 suggests that additional personnel would not appreciably decrease patient waiting time at a certain point.

Planning for Change

As mentioned previously, the process of Plan, Do, Check, Act is an excellent tool to ensure success.

- **Plan:** Goals and methods to achieve them.
  Goals:
  · Make comparison films available.
  · Optimize use of technologists.
  · Minimize reading time.
  · Measure effects of new policy.
  · Plan for contingencies.
  Methods:
  · Revise film checkout policy to allow checkout after the exam is completed.
  · Draft optimization plan to respond to peak patient load.
  · Administrator and chief radiologist review new policies with technologists, file room and reception personnel, and radiologists.
  · Administrator, reception and file room personnel, technologists, and radiologists design method to measure patient waiting time.
  · Administrator, chief technologist, and chief radiologist establish contingency plans for insufficient staffing.
- **Do:** Train and make the change.
  · *Training:* Train reception and file room personnel, technologists, and radiologists in new measurement, staffing, and film checkout policies.

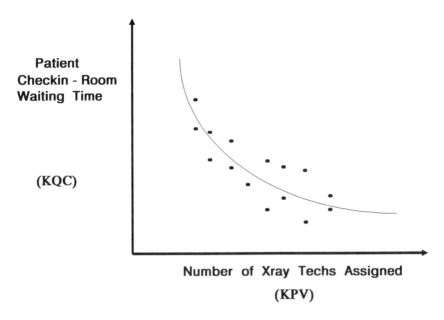

**Patient
Checkin - Room
Waiting Time**

(KQC)

**Number of Xray Techs Assigned
(KPV)**

Figure 8.9 Scatter Diagram

· *Do it:* Set implementation date with concurrence of all involved.
- **Check:** Check the effects of implementation. How many patients were studied during the previous month? What were the waiting times? How many times was it necessary to use extra personnel? Check the causes of the problems. Were there any complaints about the new procedures? Were extra personnel needed to meet the demand? How many were needed?
- **Act:** Take appropriate action based on the findings.

A note regarding Check and Act. In the journey of continuous improvement, special and system causes of variation must be thoroughly investigated. A good example was provided in Figure 8.3. Recall that when excessive patient waiting time was studied, a significant decrease resulted. In the ensuing month, however, the average time increased. This was probably due to at least two causes: (1) statistical variation and (2) failure of management to check on the changes to ensure they were being implemented.

It is remarkable how changes in methods are "translated" into processes that do not quite match the original intent. The changes that a department undergoes in the improvement process and the various "translations" of the new methods are usually not the result of people undermining the process, but are simply due to "filtering" based on individual perceptions of how the world should work (in this case the patient flow process). Such a breakdown in communication is more a reflection of the training process than a problem with workers. The need for adequate training, checking, and follow-up cannot be overemphasized.

The results over a 7-month period (Figure 8.10) showed a slight variation around the average waiting time as expected, with a slight improvement which is probably statistically insignificant. However, a noticeable improvement occurred in a decrease in the standard deviation. This is normally expected when first examining a system. The causes of variation become apparent and can be reduced.

Do such mediocre results over a 6-month period of time constitute evidence of failure in implementing TQM? Probably not, but the results would appear to be of little benefit to those seeking "instant pudding." In many cases, it will take years to perfect the method and demonstrate statistically significant results. The most important feature of this exercise was that individual workers gathered the data and made decisions to improve the problems identified.

Once the process comes under tighter control, focus can shift to issues that may result in breakthroughs, with significant reductions in waiting times. Japan did not rise from the ashes of World War II in 6 months. It took 20 years. Persevere.

REDUCING REPORT TURNAROUND TIME

Another facility identified report turnaround time as a major problem. The medical staff indicated that the time from performing the exam to the appearance of the report on the chart was too long. This information was obtained from a survey of medical staff, which highlighted several areas of dissatisfaction. Report turnaround, however, was easily the winner.

A pilot study determined that the average report turnaround time was over 48 hours. Outpatient reports averaged over 3 days, inpatient reports were in excess of 30 hours, and reports for ICU patients over 24 hours. Clearly, decisions were being made without the benefit of the radiologist's interpretation or decisions were being delayed.

The department leadership, who had all been trained in the philosophy and tools of TQM, asked the section heads (transcription, radiologists, technologists, clerks) who had an impact on generation of reports to join in defining the problem and developing an opportunity statement. In discussing the problem, it became clear that not only was report

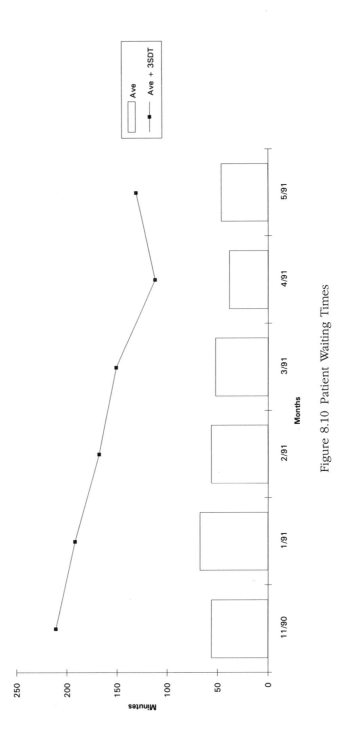

Figure 8.10 Patient Waiting Times

delivery and timely posting a problem, but it was creating a bigger problem in the reception area, file room, and reading room when referring physicians called for results. Time usually devoted to registering patients, filing films, and interpreting exams was spent transferring calls, looking up results, pulling films for re-interpretation, and re-evaluating the exams so that the physician would have the information necessary to make a therapeutic decision. Another problem became obvious during the discussion: no one from the file room had been invited to participate. This was corrected at the next meeting.

The opportunity statement was as follows:

> An opportunity exists to reduce the time it takes to generate and distribute a report, beginning with the time of the exam and ending with the time the report appears on the chart. The current process is inefficient, and referring physicians, file clerks, receptionists, and radiologists are dissatisfied because of the time required to track down the reports or the studies, re-interpret them, and transmit a report a second time. Improvement will result in reports being on the charts when needed by the physicians for decision making. A secondary improvement will be improved efficiency for file clerks, receptionists, referring physicians, and radiologists.

Let's dissect this statement.

> An opportunity exists to reduce the time it takes to generate and distribute a report, beginning with the time of the exam and ending with the time the report appears on the chart.

This states the mission of the team (reduce report turnaround time) and sets the boundaries (exam time and time until report is on the chart).

> The current process is inefficient, and referring physicians, file clerks, receptionists, and radiologists are dissatisfied because of the time required to track down the reports or the studies, re-interpret them, and transmit a report a second time.

This defines the symptoms of the problem in measurable terms (time to gather reports already done) and the impact of each.

> Improvement will result in reports being on the charts when needed by the physicians for decision making. A secondary improvement will be improved efficiency for file clerks, receptionists, referring physicians, and radiologists.

This defines the results that are expected from the improvement (reports on charts when needed—the internal customer's need).

Note once again that there is no attempt to affix blame or imply root causes or solutions. The result is sufficiently defined to allow for continuous improvement because a specific goal has not been defined.

Team Selection

The team was composed of volunteers and those asked to participate based on their knowledge and the criterion that their position within the organization affected the reporting process. Membership included a radiologist, a technologist, a transcriptionist, a receptionist, a file room clerk, and the department administrator. The administrator was elected team leader.

The team found that the opportunity statement was too broad and exceeded the departmental boundaries of control. Responsibility for entering the reports on the charts was clearly outside the area of responsibility of the radiology department. Outpatient reports were charted by the individual doctors' offices and inpatient reports were charted by ward secretaries.

The opportunity statement was revised to read "distributed and available" instead of "on the chart."

Identifying the Reporting Process

The team defined the process as outlined in the report turnaround time flowchart (Figure 8.11). The major steps in reporting were identified as exam production, exam presentation, interpretation, transcription, and report distribution.

This team decided to gather data on each of the steps to identify the greatest problems. The following data were selected:

- Date and time of exam
- Date and time exam read
- Date and time report transcribed
- Date and time report distributed

Obvious Improvements

Several obvious improvements were identified. A substantial number of reports were left over from the previous evening to be transcribed the following morning. Completing all transcription the same day resulted in some reduction in average turnaround time.

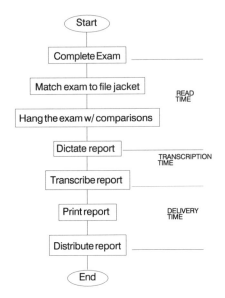

Figure 8.11 Report Turnaround Flowchart

Reports printed late in the day were not distributed until the following morning. Distributing the reports at the end of each shift also reduced the average turnaround time.

Measuring Time

An existing reporting standard required that the date and time of the exam, dictation, and transcription appear on all reports. The remaining information could be obtained by date/time stamping the reports sampled for the project. A random sample of 160 to 200 reports was found to provide a relatively accurate picture of the true turnaround time per measurement period.

The project was accomplished as follows:

- **Plan:** Goals and methods to achieve them.
  - *Goals:* Achieve a baseline average and standard deviation for elapsed time from exam to dictation, dictation to transcription, and transcription to delivery.
  - *Methods:* Team members from transcription and delivery were to randomly gather ten reports each working day. These reports were to be entered into a database from which averages and standard deviations could be calculated monthly.

- **Do:** Little education was necessary because those conducting the study had designed it. Implementation was simply conducting the study. It was agreed that the study would be completed before the next monthly meeting.
- **Check:** The team leader confirmed that reports were being randomly selected and entered in the database and were being checked for causes of problems. Interestingly, the study also pointed out which of the radiologists were conforming to the reporting standard. Improved compliance resulted from simply providing the radiologists with feedback on the compliance rates and the impact on the turnaround project.
- **Act:** The team had the information needed to pursue improvement.

While the team worked on the flowchart and determined the supplier, input, output, action, customer relationships, members also gathered the above data. It had previously been determined that this information would be needed when the team was ready to focus on quality characteristics and process variables.

The team expected to take 4 weeks to reach this point and therefore set a goal of sampling 7 to 10 reports at random each working day for the next month. This would provide a database of 187 reports by the time the information was needed.

The benchmarks established for the project are shown in control chart format in Figure 8.12. Subsequent measurements would be plotted on these control charts to (1) identify report times that exceed the upper control limits and (2) evaluate trends that may show increased or decreased turnaround times.

Finding the Hang-Ups

The Pareto chart in Figure 8.13 indicates the major contributors to increased report turnaround time. Time to interpretation was obviously the first to tackle, followed closely by transcription. The flowchart required some additional detail in this area.

Information-Based Decision Making

Focusing on time to interpretation as a key quality characteristic, the process variables that contributed to delays were displayed in a fishbone diagram (Figure 8.14). The greatest contributor to increased time to interpretation was the process of matching many of the films done in the afternoon and hanging them after the radiologist had departed for the day, which built in at least a 13-hour delay.

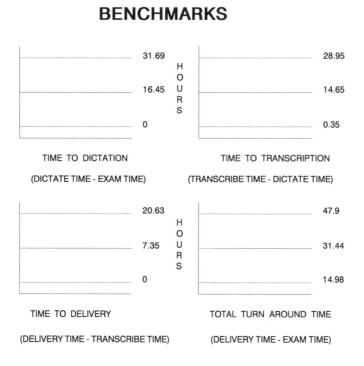

Figure 8.12 Turnaround Time Control Charts

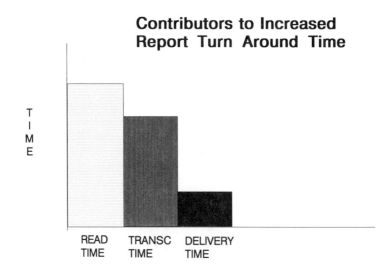

Figure 8.13 Pareto Chart

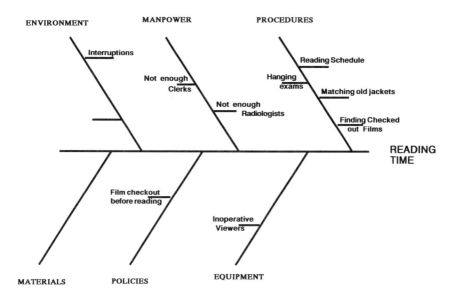

Figure 8.14 Cause-and-Effect Diagram

The importance of timely completion of the studies was not lost on the radiologists whose contracts were up for review by the hospital. Work schedules were adjusted to allow completion of all work by the end of the day, which resulted in a decrease in average report turn-around time.

The contribution of transcription was more complicated. In evaluating this segment of the process, the following information was discovered:

1. There was little for the transcriptionists to do early in the day because the radiologists were busy accomplishing scheduled procedures.
2. There was a massive amount of transcription to accomplish at the end of the normal working day because most of the dictations were done in the afternoon.

A histogram (Figure 8.15) of the dictation workload showed that in order for transcription to keep up with the workload, fewer typists were needed in the morning and more were needed in the afternoon.

Planning for Change

Discussions between the radiologists and the transcriptionists were initiated, with the chief radiologist and lead transcriptionist supporting

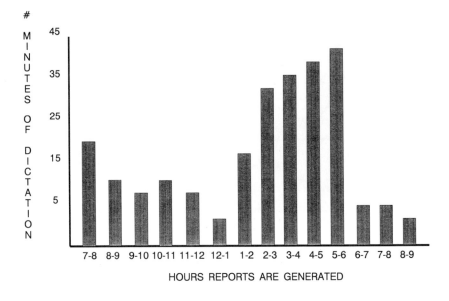

Figure 8.15 Histogram of Reports Generated

the improvement project. By reviewing the purpose and mission of the department and focusing on customer satisfaction as the driving interest, the interested parties realized that an adjustment in working hours would facilitate a marked improvement in report turnaround time.

All personnel impacted by the change were consulted. Plans were made to change the work hours, effective several weeks in the future.

Making It Happen

Once the changes were in place, sampling of random reports was resumed. As expected, the averages were reduced. Attention was then directed to the next area that was the greatest contributor to report turnaround time (distribution).

IMPROVING PATIENT ACCESS

One facility wanted to decrease the backlog of scheduled exams and increase volume and at the same time improve patient access. They wanted to do this intelligently, with a good business plan in mind. The hospital had determined that patients were going to a rival facility with a shorter wait for scheduled exams.

This is certainly a more complex issue than the preceding examples. It illustrates that as the continuous improvement journey progresses, problem solving may become more complex but remains achievable through the use of TQM.

Finding Barriers to Patient Access

This facility flowcharted the process of delivering scheduled examinations. One area had a backlog of scheduled exams. By maintaining close contacts with the medical staff offices, it was determined that patients were being sent to a competing facility where the exams could be scheduled earlier.

A look at the schedule showed the backlog for exams to be 1 1/2 weeks. The referring physicians preferred examinations within 3 days. The opportunity statement read as follows:

> An opportunity exists to improve access of patients to the radiology department, beginning with the scheduling of the patients and ending with the examination completed within a time frame acceptable to the referring physicians.
>
> The current system results in lost business and loss of market share and potentially loss of reputation in the community.
>
> Improvement should result in a reduced number of patients being sent to competing facilities for scheduled examinations.

The team consisted of the department administrator, the chief technologist, a lead technologist, a lead receptionist, and a radiologist.

A flowchart (Figure 8.16) showed that there was no flexibility to adapt to peak loads. If the earliest available slot was not acceptable to the patient or the referring physician, the patient was not scheduled. This obviously was a mechanism to manage the workload, but it did not take advantage of the opportunity to expand the service.

Obvious Improvements

It was obvious that flexibility in the schedule was needed in order to adapt to changes in request rates. What was less obvious was how to accomplish this.

Operational Data Needed

The team first examined the present capacity. With four rooms and staffing for five days of operations and after-hours emergencies, it was obvious that if the number of patients was going to increase, one or two

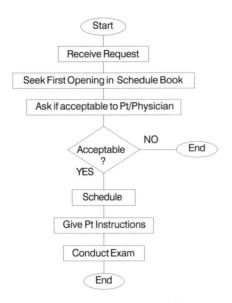

Figure 8.16 Patient Access Process

changes needed to occur: the hours (and staffing) needed to be expanded, the efficiency of conducting the exams needed to be improved, or both.

The average time for conducting each exam and preparing the room for the next exam was calculated from data obtained by measurement. The 35-minute average exam and room turnover time showed that approximately two exams could be completed each hour per room. The current schedule called for an exam slot each half hour from 7:30 a.m. to 11:30 a.m. This yielded a maximum of eight examinations per day per room. With 2 rooms available, 16 examinations per day were possible.

The time of radiologist involvement was also needed in order to assess workload capacity. Speaking to the patient, conducting the exam, and reading/dictating the exam was calculated to require 27 minutes on the average. Thus, 16 exams would require 16 × 27 or 7.2 hours (432 minutes). If this number of exams was scheduled each day, the radiologist would have time for little else.

The team next examined historical data for the maximum number of exams conducted monthly. They interviewed referring physician office staff in an attempt to estimate the number of patients that bypassed the department. The maximum number of exams completed in the recent past was 221, and an estimated 20 patients per month were being lost to other facilities due to the scheduling backlog. Thus, a maximum of 241 exams was possible during each month or a maximum of approximately 12 per day. The average number of exams was 164 per month or 8 per day.

This may seem like simple mathematics to solve the problem. However, one examination competes with other examinations scheduled at the same time using other rooms and also competes for the time of the technologists and radiologists. This situation must also be evaluated to ensure that the solution does not "rob Peter to pay Paul."

Making Operational Change Proposals

Capacity issues were addressed first. It was decided to propose an adjustment in staffing based on the average number of exams performed per day. Overtime would be paid for the additional time that would be required to complete the excess exams. The overall workload was such that the radiologists added a part-time radiologist on Saturdays to open up an additional six slots per week. This added 24 slots to the average of 164 per month, leaving 53 slots (maximum of 241 minus the revised average of 188) which could potentially be filled during normal working hours. This represented about three additional exams daily above the average schedule of eight.

Issues relating to flexibility of service were addressed next. A policy proposal was drafted which allowed the reception personnel to over-schedule up to three exams per day whenever a request was received and the next three days were full. Reception personnel would also notify the chief technologist and chief radiologist whenever over-scheduling occurred.

The proposal to the hospital administration included the variable costs of the plan:

Estimated revenue:	53 × $170	=	$9010
Estimated overtime:	53 × 0.5 hrs × $21	=	($557)
Total additional revenue:			$8453

The professional cost was minimal in that the overall increased workload outside fluoro justified an additional part-time radiologist.

Implementing Operational Change

- **Plan:** Goals and methods to achieve them.
  Goals:
  · Change schedule.
  · Change scheduling policy.

  · Change method of determining when exam results are needed.
  · Measure effects of new policy.
  · Plan for contingencies.
  Methods:
  · Receptionists create schedule form.
  · Receptionists and administrator draft new policy.
  · Administrator and chief radiologist review new policy with technologists and radiologists.
  · Administrator and reception personnel design method for measuring number of patients referred elsewhere.
  · Administrator, chief technologist, and chief radiologist establish plans for sufficient staffing
- **Do:** Train and make the change.
  · *Training:* Train reception personnel, technologists, and radiologists in new scheduling and exam performance policies.
  · *Do it:* Set implementation date with concurrence of all involved.
- **Check:** Check the effects of implementation. How many patients were examined during the previous month? How many were referred elsewhere? How many times was it necessary to over-schedule? Were there any complaints about the new procedures? Was temporary help needed to meet the demand? How much help was needed?
- **Act**: Take appropriate action based on the findings.

SOLVING REVENUE PROBLEMS

A facility wanted to show that TQM indeed resulted in savings or increased revenue. They decided to examine coding as a possible source of error in denied claims.

Total denied claims from third-party payers was in excess of $100,000 during one quarter. The leading cause of the denials was incorrect ICD-9 codes.

The Coding Process

The coding process was fairly simple, as shown in Figure 8.17. Obvious improvements were not readily apparent at this point. What was apparent was that the internal supplier in the coding process could be the radiologist and the internal customer could be the coding specialist. The radiologists had never considered that they could be part of the collection problem.

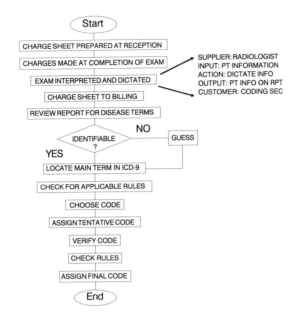

Figure 8.17 Billing/Coding Process

Finding Variability in Collections

In determining the needs and expectations of the customers (coding specialists), the radiologists found that the coding specialists needed assistance in determining why an exam was conducted or what underlying disease was being evaluated (ruled out/in). The radiographic reports frequently failed to yield such information and the medical records were not readily available to the coding specialists.

In identifying causes by brainstorming and adding three potential causes to the fishbone diagram (Figure 8.18), it was found that, from the perspective of the radiologists, insufficient clinical information was provided by the clinicians. However, the technologists were good at asking the patients why they were being examined, and more than 90% of the time they could determine a reasonable patient history that would result in a tentative diagnosis. It was also pointed out to the radiologists that the issue of referring physicians not providing adequate clinical information was moot in that the loss of professional radiologist fees was not the concern of the clinicians. If the radiologists wanted to improve collections, they would have to adopt the position of satisfying their customers (the coding specialist and the insurance company) by providing sufficient patient data to allow for appropriate payment.

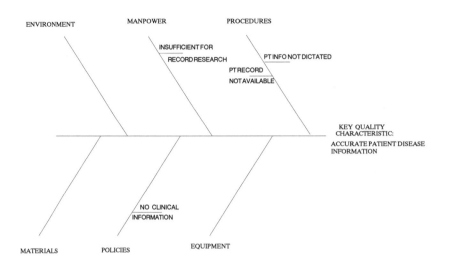

Figure 8.18 Fishbone Diagram of Cause and Effect

Operational Changes to Improve Collections

Evaluation of a sampling of denied claims indicated that if the radiologists had added to their reports the brief clinical information that was available with the requisition, more than 80% of the claims would probably have been paid. This would have resulted in an increase of approximately $70,000 in revenues during one quarter. With this information the radiologists became quick converts to the TQM process.

PITFALLS

Exceeding the boundaries of the task: Improvement teams that exceed their areas of control may offend those responsible for the operation of those areas. Also, lack of authority to change processes in these areas may lead to frustration. At first, improvement projects should be restricted to areas within the authority of the department. These boundaries may be exceeded only with the approval and cooperation of those whose areas the boundaries cross.

Not defining boundaries of responsibility: This is similar to exceeding the boundaries. The purpose of the team, as well as the boundaries of their charge, must be clear.

Reacting to mistakes made by the improvement team: Nothing will stop the momentum of the improvement process more than reacting negatively to mistakes. An atmosphere must be created in which those involved in the effort can speak freely about their mistakes and observations. To prevent recurrences, all involved in the effort must discuss the problems.

Do not entertain the excuse "I don't know": A more appropriate response in the improvement effort would be "Let's find out using by the tools of TQM."

Failure to follow up on actions: This will result in maintaining the status quo. Be sure to check and recheck to ensure that the education is appropriate and the new processes are being implemented properly. There will always be the 10% who do not quite get it right the first time.

Making decisions with incomplete or erroneous information: Failure to exhaust all the possible causes that may contribute to a problem may result in choosing the wrong thing to fix. We all have a tendency to see order where none exists. Carefully constructed questions are necessary to ensure that the information obtained is fair and balanced and does not just support the hypothesis. An adequate sample is another requirement in making decisions based on statistics. The need to obtain the services of a reputable statistician cannot be overemphasized.

Obvious improvements that have a negative impact: This indicates that all the criteria for an obvious improvement were not considered or that the flowchart may not be an accurate portrayal of the process.

Dealing with setbacks: This is usually the result of normal statistical variation. Remain focused on the vision and mission of the department with knowledge of the guiding principles. Recall from Chapter 7 the discussion of early exhilaration and the frustration of realizing that total quality requires effort, coupled with the discomfort of an incomplete understanding of and a lack of experience in utilizing the tools of TQM. Focus on education of the improvement teams and they will succeed.

9

IMPROVEMENT in
DIAGNOSIS and THERAPEUTICS

When an organization dwells exclusively on finding, blaming, and rooting out deficient individuals, departments, or disciplines, its attention is also diverted away from the essential need to measure, assess, and improve everyday processes, systems, and functions.

The Measurement Mandate
JCAHO

Some physicians consider themselves independent of the healthcare system that supports their efforts. In order to successfully implement improvement efforts, the physician must realize that he or she is a part (albeit a significant part) of the healthcare system and must participate in studying the system in which he or she works. The purpose of this chapter is to demonstrate that the clinical aspects of radiologic practice can indeed be studied using the tools of Total Quality Management (TQM) and improvement can be achieved as a result.

One of the major hurdles in implementing a program such as TQM is gaining the confidence of the physicians and obtaining their cooperation. Similar to the description of change in Chapter 7, some physician leaders will readily see the benefit of TQM and become early proponents. Most, however, will adopt a "wait and see" attitude. The following steps are recommended in winning over the medical staff: (1) educate the physicians as to the difference between TQM and Quality Assurance (QA), (2) appeal to the reasons they entered the practice of medicine and to the scientific method of quality improvement, (3) demonstrate practical applications, and as a last resort (4) show them how it can affect their revenue (as in the last example in Chapter 8).

Some of the aspects of applying the principles of TQM to the clinical practice of diagnostic radiology will be discussed in this chapter. To begin, it is critical to determine how radiology fits into the healthcare system. Dr. David Eddy concisely defined the essence of clinical quality improvement by stating that the quality of medical care is determined by (1) the quality of the decisions that determine what actions are taken and (2) the quality with which those actions are carried out. Both medical decision making and the acceptability of the actions that are performed can be measured by capturing appropriate pieces of information. It is the premise of this chapter that (1) the quality of information provided by radiology has an impact on the quality of medical decisions made and (2) the acceptability of actions and guidance by the radiologist have an impact on the outcome of patient care.

IMPROVING BREAST CANCER DETECTION

The Detection Process

Breast cancer screening differs somewhat from the diagnostic model provided in Chapter 6. In screening programs, asymptomatic patients are studied to ascertain the presence of disease that would otherwise go undetected until clinically apparent.

The process of detection includes the subprocess of exam production (acceptable positioning of the patient's breast on the film cassette, acceptable exposure of the film, acceptable processing of the film, and acceptable matching of the current exam with old exam for comparison) and the subprocess of exam interpretation. Bear in mind that even though the subprocess of exam production is considered outside the interpretive efforts of the radiologist, the radiologist is responsible for ensuring that the procedures listed above are indeed acceptable.

Detection also depends on the skill of the radiologist to detect an abnormality and correctly interpret its relationship to the presence or absence of breast cancer. This is a complex function of the radiologist's training, fund of knowledge, and reading environment and the incidence of breast cancer within the population served.

There is considerable room for variation in both production and interpretation. Variation is usually found in exposures, positioning, and the radiologist's knowledge base. The American College of Radiology's Accreditation Program has done a superb job of providing standardization for breast screening in the United States. However, accreditation cannot compensate for training. This is a function of PDCA and must be carried out as a routine part of the operation of the department.

The focus of the next section is the accuracy and consistency of interpretations and efforts that may be undertaken to improve them.

Find a Problem

In one facility, referring physicians complained that one radiologist would tell them one thing and another would tell them something else. Some referring physicians would not discuss mammograms with several of the radiologists, because they lacked confidence in their interpretations. Scheduling difficulties resulted, because mammograms from some requesting physicians had to be read by certain radiologists who may have had other duties assigned.

In a sampling of mammographic cases for peer review, it was confirmed that there was considerable variation in interpreting exams. Further sampling indicated that some radiologists failed to provide adequate interpretations and follow-up recommendations using the current literature as the standard for mammographic reports. The most frequent complaint was that findings described on the report did not include recommendations as to what to the referring physician should do or what the findings meant. No recommendations were offered for additional examinations that would improve diagnostic certainty. Many breast cancers were detected, but minimal cancers were not.

Faced with this data, the radiologists agreed to participate in the improvement process. Increasing competition for patients and the need for a high-quality product served as incentives to encourage participation.

The opportunity statement reads as follows:

An opportunity exists to improve the quality of mammographic interpretations and reports by reducing the variation among radiologists and by establishing standards for reporting. The present system creates confusion among the referring physicians. The routine whereby referring physicians review mammograms with other radiologists as a result of lack of confidence in some radiologists wastes time for both the radiologists and the referring physicians. The stage of cancer at detection may potentially be elevated by this variation. Improvement should result in reduced variation in interpretations and fewer disagreements in peer review. Improved earlier detection of breast cancer may result in the long term.

Organize a Team

A team of radiologists was formed to tackle the problem. The team included the radiologists who demonstrated a need for improvement. It was preferable for them to participate in making the change rather than having it imposed upon them.

Clarify the Problem

In clarifying the problem, the team first had to define what they were going to measure in order to accomplish the task of reducing variation in mammographic interpretations. The improvement model does not change, because this is clinical medicine rather than departmental logistics. There is a process to the interpretation of all exams if one gives it some thought. The flowchart documenting the process is shown in Figure 9.1.

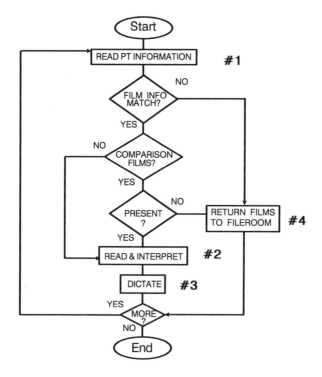

Figure 9.1 Interpretation Process

In defining the basic processes (Figure 9.2) for reading and interpretation, it became clear that the radiologist was the supplier who provided an input (mammographic knowledge and skill) to the action (read and interpret the mammogram) which produced an output (mammographic report) for a customer (referring physician and patient). Other customers defined for the record were the transcriptionist who transcribed the reports and the data gatherers who entered the patient data into the mammogram database (these are logistic functions and will not be covered here in order to concentrate on the clinical aspects of mammographic improvement).

The needs and expectations of the customers (patients and referring physicians) were determined by asking them what they wanted in mammography:

1. A highly accurate report
2. Consistency among the radiologists
3. Recommendations for follow-up examinations
4. A concise and clear report with consistent terminology

Understanding the Problem

In brainstorming the causes of variation in interpretations which did not satisfy the first three needs and expectations (report accuracy and consistency and follow-up recommendations), the team relied on their experience in peer review of mammograms. A number of factors that contributed to variation were identified, and by using multivoting several were selected as the most influential:

1. Out-of-date knowledge base
2. Lack of agreement on terminology
3. Lack of agreement on criteria for malignant vs. benign
4. Lack of agreement on workup of indeterminate
5. Lack of appreciation for a screening program
6. Lack of consistent terminology

These causes were graphically displayed in a fishbone diagram (Figure 9.3A) as well as a Pareto chart (Figure 9.3B), with the most significant receiving the most votes. Another way to determine the most significant causes is to tabulate the number of times peer review revealed a discrepancy and categorize by cause. One pitfall to avoid is studying a problem to the detriment of what is to be accomplished (otherwise known as studying a problem to death). Common sense prevails in many venues and works in quality improvement as well.

PROCESS WORKSHEET: Define the basic processes in the flowchart						
Proc #	Supplier	Input	Action	Output	Customer	Needs and Expectations
#2	RADs	Knowledge Skill	Interpretation	Opinion	1. Referring Physician 2. Patient	1. Clear, Concise, Accurate, and Timely report with follow up recommendations. 2. Clear, Concise, Accurate, and Timely report with follow up recommendations.
#3	RADs	Knowledge Skill	Dictation	Voice Record	Transcription	Clear, Concise dictation.

Figure 9.2 Process Worksheet

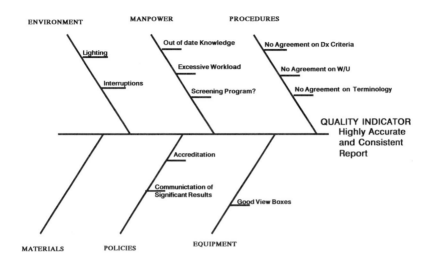

Figure 9.3A Cause-and-Effect Diagram

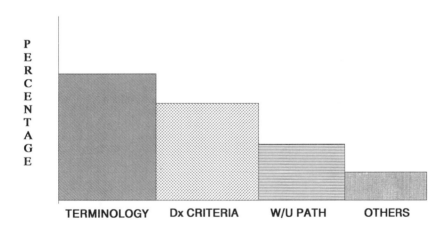

Figure 9.3B Contributors to Report Variation

There is usually no real need to prove the obvious. However, the obvious can sometimes be shown to be wrong, and this can only be revealed by studying the problem in greater detail.

Selecting the Best Current Solution

Before work could begin on items 3 and 4 (criteria and workup recommendations), it was clear that the team would need some education in the latest knowledge about breast disease, terminology, and the purpose and definitions of a screening program. Therefore, members were scheduled for continuing medical education (CME) in breast disease, the current literature was reviewed for the latest information, and the breast imaging lexicon of the American College of Radiology was adopted as the basis for consistent terminology. Simultaneously, work began on defining measures of effectiveness in mammographic detection of breast disease and establishing benchmarks against which the effect of using these criteria could be assessed.

Once education was complete, criteria for malignancy and benign were selected, followed by selection of criteria for follow-up of any examination considered to be indeterminate.

What followed was part of the continuous cycle of Plan, Do, Check, Act (PDCA):

1. **Plan:** Schedule CME. Plan pertinent literature search. Learn ACR lexicon of Breast Imaging Reporting And Data System (BIRADS).
   Do: Provide CME. Search literature and assign articles to be read. Review ACR lexicon.
   Check: Accomplished?
   Act: Begin selecting criteria and recommended workups.
2. **Plan:** Choose measurement method to evaluate the outcome of mammographic interpretations.
   Do: Begin data collection and entry for benchmark values.
   Check: Evaluate the integrity of the data.
   Act: Use benchmarks to determine improvement.
3. **Plan:** Choose measurement method to evaluate the use of the criteria developed.
   Do: Measure use of the criteria.
   Check: Are the criteria being used? Are referring physicians satisfied with the reports?
   Act: Reinforce use or adjust as necessary.
4. **Plan:** Continue measurement method to evaluate the outcome of mammographic interpretations.
   Do: Continue data collection and entry.

Check: Evaluate the integrity of the data. When the database is sufficiently large, evaluate exam characteristics.

Act: Respond to findings as appropriate.

Data Collection

A mammogram database was developed to run on personal computers placed in the mammography suites of the hospital mammography units. The following data were collected:

Patient ID info	Follow-up recommendations
Clinical Info	Film QC
Doctor info	Bx/Surg results
Radiologist info	TP/FP/TN/FN
Tech info	Cancer stage
Exam date	Localization info
Mammo findings	

In order to demonstrate improvement, whatever is to be improved must be quantifiable in some fashion. Areas in mammography that can be quantified include the predictive values of breast biopsy recommendations, the false-negative interpretation rate, the proportion of breast cancer patients distributed by stage of cancer at diagnosis, the percent of patients recommended for short-term follow-up, and the percent of screening patients brought back for diagnostic studies. This should not be considered an exhaustive list, but it does provide the basics of a screening program to evaluate effectiveness.

In addition, the team developed a registry of information to be maintained on their mammogram patients in order to provide long-term information about the quality of the mammography product. The information was designed to assess the adequacy of breast cancer detection. Statistics were obtained to determine the positive breast cancer biopsy rate, the rate at which screening patients were referred for diagnostic mammograms, and a comparison of the rates relative to one another categorized by interpreting radiologist. Localization failure rates were also computed, and film quality was assessed by the same database. Cancer stage at diagnosis was also collected for the population.

Analysis

Caution must be exercised in that results should not be judged solely on the basis of such data as listed above. Many confounding aspects can influence outcomes such as positive biopsy rates. For example, a largely Medicare population may allow for a higher positive biopsy rate, while a predominately younger screening population may have a much lower positive biopsy rate. Future improvement efforts may evaluate the positive biopsy rate (positive predictive value—surgical) as a function of cancer stage, patient age at detection, or breast type.

Two well-known theories of breast cancer screening are that the predictive value of biopsy recommendations will likely (1) increase with the age of the patient and (2) decrease with an increasing percentage of minimal breast cancer detection (the price of early detection is a decreased biopsy positive predictive value). These theories are illustrated in Figures 9.4A and B, where the predictive values are plotted against patient age and cancer stage at detection. Cancer stage has been shown to more accurately predict patient outcome than the size or tissue grade of the tumor and is therefore used as a yardstick for effectiveness of outcome.

The database developed by this facility also allowed for stratification of these data by patient age and breast types to evaluate sources of diagnostic difficulties and test the theories. Once again, TQM allows for the formulation of theories against which the data are tested in order to support or deny the theory.

Consulting with a statistician is strongly recommended when designing data collection for clinical purposes. Time can be saved and useful information collected by employing someone who can improve the likelihood of obtaining meaningful data and analyzing it.

An article by Dr. Edward Sickles ("Quality Assurance." *Radiologic Clinics of North America*, pp. 265–275, January 1992) is recommended for further information on quality audits in mammography.

Making Improvement Continuous

In fulfilling the purpose of the department to provide improved diagnostic effectiveness and fulfilling the purpose of the team (which should be in line with the purpose of the department) to improve patient outcomes, the team may want to direct its efforts toward maximizing detection of low-stage cancers and minimizing detection of high-stage disease (Figure 9.5). At the same time, however, it is important that this is not accomplished at the risk of over-biopsying the screening population.

The most important aspect of continuous improvement is that it be integrated into the daily routine of practicing radiology. It should not be considered as something over and above the process of image interpretation, but rather should be considered a part of doing business. The true results of such an undertaking will take years to realize. The important thing is that steps are taken now for future improvement.

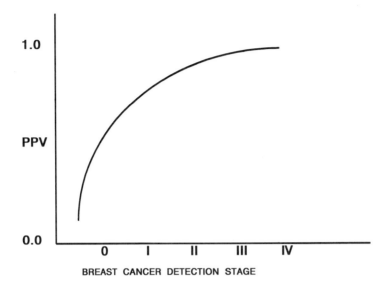

Figure 9.4A Predictive Value vs. Cancer Stage

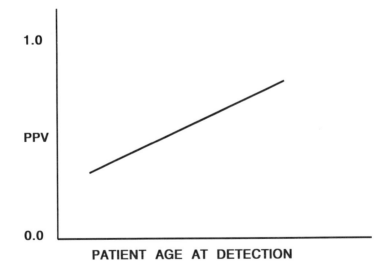

Figure 9.4B Predictive Value vs. Age at Detection

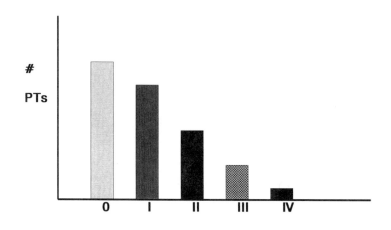

Figure 9.5 Breast Cancer Screening Detection Stage

OPTIMIZING MAGNETIC RESONANCE DIAGNOSIS

Quality Control of Image Acquisition

A number of methods are available to maintain the quality of the images produced. The bad news is that there are many. The good news is that service contracts usually provide for maintenance of the factors that will be briefly discussed in this section. These factors include center resonant frequency, image uniformity, spatial linearity, high contrast spatial resolution, slice thickness, and minimizing image artifacts. Technologists should have a working knowledge of these factors to assist in detecting and correcting image problems, whether the correction is actually made by the technologist or the service engineer.

Resonant Frequency

The center resonant frequency should be measured daily and compared with previous results. The measurements can be plotted on a control chart (Figure 9.6A). The center frequency f_0 for hydrogen is 42.58 MHz/T. For example, a 1.5-Tesla system should operate at 1.5 × 42.58 = 63.87 MHz. Variation greater than 50 ppm or a trend of 4 or more points from the resonant frequency should result in a search for the cause.

Variables that affect center resonant frequency are displayed in a fishbone diagram in Figure 9.6B.

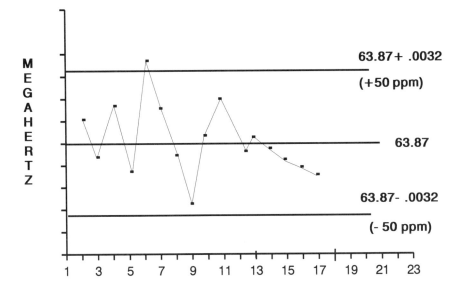

Figure 9.6A Frequency Control Chart

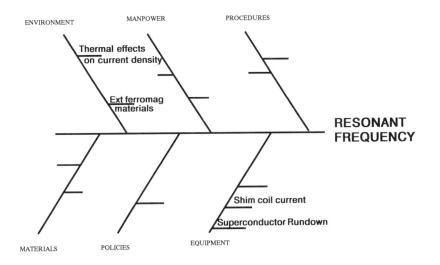

Figure 9.6B Fishbone Diagram of Cause and Effect

Image Uniformity

Uniformity of the signal intensity over the scanned volume is essential to distinguishing normal from abnormal. This is measured by scanning a volume with homogeneous MR characteristics (phantom). Image uniformity (Figure 9.7A) should be in excess of 80% for a field of view of 20 cm or less imaged with a body coil (Figure 9.7B).

Variables that affect uniformity are displayed in a fishbone diagram in Figure 9.7C.

Spatial Linearity

Spatial linearity is related to geometrical distortion in that a displayed point is located away from its position in the slice volume of the specimen. It is calculated by measuring the distance between two points on the image and the true distance in the imaging volume and comparing them (Figure 9.8A). Linearity should be less than 5% in a field of view greater than 25 cm (Figure 9.8B).

Variables that affect linearity are displayed in Figure 9.8C.

Slice Thickness

Slice thickness can be defined as either the full width at half maximum (as in nuclear medicine) or full width at one tenth maximum (Figure 9.9A). The measured slice thickness should be within +1 mm for slices greater than 5 mm (Figure 9.9B).

Contributing variables are indicated in Figure 9.9C.

Imaging Artifacts

Imaging artifacts are usually due to phase-related "ghosting" or unusually high or low signal intensity where it is not expected. The most common source of phase-related artifacts is motion by the patient. These artifacts are most effectively dealt with by the knowledgeable MR radiologist selecting appropriate phase encoding directions to "throw" the artifact off the areas of interest.

Other artifacts are the result of quadrature coil phase errors. A summary of causes is provided in Figure 9.10.

The MR Knowledge Base

This is strictly based on individual capability, but variability within a group can be reduced by reaching consensus on criteria and creating checklists of items that should be addressed for each type of exam. However, because the field of magnetic resonance imaging is virtually

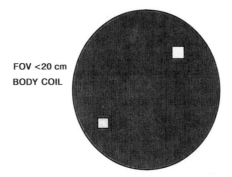

Figure 9.7A Image Uniformity

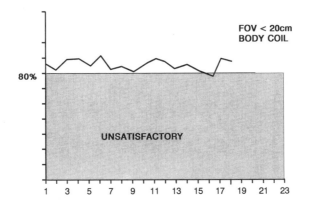

Figure 9.7B Image Uniformity

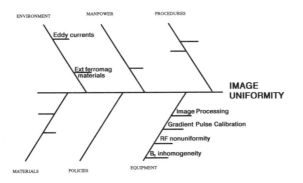

Figure 9.7C Fishbone Diagram of Cause and Effect

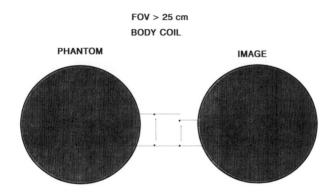

Figure 9.8A Spatial Linearity

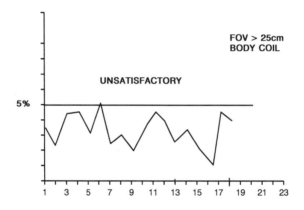

Figure 9.8B Spatial Linearity

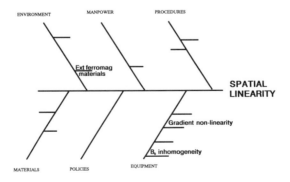

Figure 9.8C Fishbone Diagram of Cause and Effect

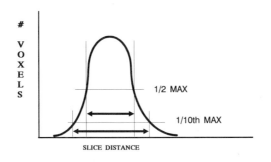

Figure 9.9A Measuring Slice Thickness

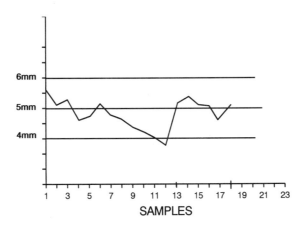

Figure 9.9B Slice Thickness Control Chart

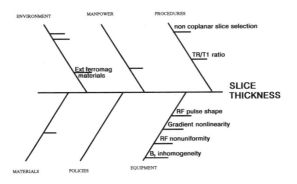

Figure 9.9C Fishbone Diagram of Cause and Effect

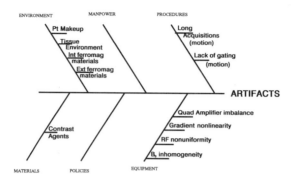

Figure 9.10 Fishbone Diagram of Cause and Effect

exploding with new pulse sequences and capabilities, the checklist of criteria should be regularly updated to reflect the current capability of the system.

Choosing the Right "Gold" Standard

Any improvement effort should include the feedback loop of tissue proof weighed against the interpretation and differential diagnosis offered in the report. The source of the "gold" standard used must be taken into consideration in determining sensitivity, specificity, and predictive values. A reliable pathology department is essential, particularly in cytology if fine needle aspirations are to be used as the source. Additionally, arthroscopic findings are highly dependent upon the skill of the arthroscopist.

CROSS-FUNCTIONAL IMPROVEMENT PROGRAMS

A future expectation of accreditation bodies and healthcare reform in general is to extend improvement beyond departmental boundaries. This endorses the idea that the customer (patient) experiences not only the effects of an encounter with the radiology department, but also has an encounter with the institution in which the department is located. How the radiology department interacts with the many other activities within a hospital or medical center will determine not only the success of the department but the success of the institution as well.

Examples of such an experience may be found is the diagnosis of pulmonary embolus (PE). This is obviously a multi-specialty and multi-modality diagnostic pathway; it may originate with an orthopedic surgeon who consults with an internist who consults with nuclear medicine and potentially an angiographer. Consider a hospital in which PE may be under-diagnosed because physicians are unwilling to perform or request pulmonary angiography. Another scenario may be due to reluctance to perform and request pulmonary angiography, where patients with this suspected diagnosis are shunted to another facility or are transferred in order to obtain the proper workup.

Such was the case at one facility. A review of the current literature and standards revealed that the diagnostic workup fell short of the standard of care expected. A problem was identified (Found), and the opportunity statement was drafted as follows:

> An opportunity exists to improve the diagnostic certainty of pulmonary embolus. The current workup does not follow the currently recommended diagnostic routines, resulting in a possible increase in morbidity or loss of occupied bed days if the patient is transferred. Improvement should result in improved diagnostic certainty, improved treatment, decreased morbidity, and increased reimbursable occupied bed days.

A team was assembled (Organized) to address the issue. A vascular surgeon, a pulmonologist, a radiologist, and a nuclear medicine specialist formed the initial team. A review of the current literature and the diagnostic armamentarium was conducted and a diagnostic pathway was proposed.

There was strong reluctance on the part of the medical staff to follow up an indeterminate probability of PE on a nuclear medicine scan. The clinicians would decide whether or not to treat based solely on their clinical impressions. Thus, some patients were subjected to the risks of thrombolytic therapy or were diagnosed with PE without a measured diagnostic certainty. The medical leaders wanted to change this to improve the certainty of diagnosis for PE.

A measure of morbidity was defined as any untoward event that occurred during the hospitalization of a patient with a diagnosis of suspected PE.

Clarifying the Problem

In evaluating the diagnostic pathway, the team considered the diagnostic modalities available and the skills available at each modality.

The ability of the medical staff to accurately assess the likelihood of PE based on history, physical examination, laboratory tests, and electrocardiograms was largely unknown. Also unknown were the predictive values of the ventilation/perfusion scans, venograms, and doppler venous ultrasound.

Therefore, the diagnostic pathway (Figure 9.11) was predicated on the sensitivities and specificities found in the literature for each modality, and it was assumed that the modalities practiced at the facility were comparable to the literature. The measures to be accomplished would determine the validity of this assumption.

Understanding the Problem

A review of previous cases of suspected PE revealed that few had been worked up beyond the ventilation/perfusion scan; the few that were referred for pulmonary angiography revealed a breakdown in communication between nuclear medicine and angiography and inconsistencies in conducting the angiograms. Therefore, specific pathways were established within the radiology department to serve as a standard against which the diagnostic workup could be measured

The specific steps that the department agreed to follow in the workup of PE are presented in Figure 9.12. A micro flowchart of the angiographic procedure agreed upon by the radiologists is presented in Figure 9.13.

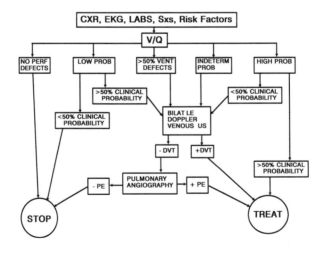

Figure 9.11 Diagnostic Pathway for Pulmonary Embolism

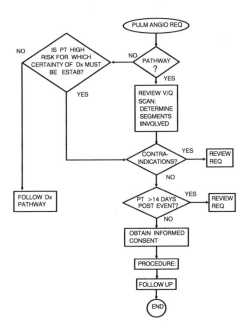

Figure 9.12 Preliminary Steps Leading to Pulmonary Angiography

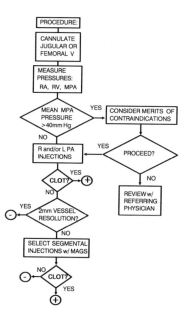

Figure 9.13 Pulmonary Arteriogram Process

In evaluating the effectiveness (recall the definition from Chapter 6) of the imaging modalities used, the team identified specific items to be measured in order to improve the diagnostic process.

Selecting the Best Current Solution

After defining the pathway to be tested, it was time to implement it and test it:

- **Plan:** The first goal was to test the pathway. Steps for implementation included (1) defining and standardizing criteria for each diagnostic modality, (2) considering the need for instruction in each modality and providing training as needed, and (3) educating medical staff in order to ensure compliance with the diagnostic pathway.

- **Do:** It was determined that it would be necessary to standardize the criteria for each diagnostic modality in order to measure the effectiveness. Diagnostic criteria were established and specific tests required as a minimum. In addition, refresher training was conducted in doppler venous ultrasound and pulmonary angiography. A target date was established for implementing the diagnostic pathway, and conferences were held with medical staff members to encourage participation.

- **Check:** Data sheets were obtained on all patients for whom the diagnosis of PE was considered to the point of requesting a ventilation/perfusion scan. Initially, the team was primarily interested in determining if there was compliance with the diagnostic pathway. This would help determine the validity of the data obtained and whether or not it was useful in diagnosing PE. An assessment of the clinical utility of the diagnostic criteria would be undertaken later.

- **Act:** The team would continue to look critically at the diagnostic pathway to determine if it served the needs of the patients and was feasible under the conditions at the facility, keeping in mind that the primary purpose of the team was to improve diagnostic certainty and treatment of disease.

THOUGHTS ON FUTURE APPLICATIONS

Looking to the future and toward the application of TQM in the radiologic setting, some of the areas to explore are as follows:

- **Exam value:** Has the exam provided improved knowledge about the patient's condition and is it useful therapeutically? Is the value equal to the cost and the quality?
- **Customer satisfaction:** What does the customer need that he or she does not expect or has not yet thought of to achieve satisfaction? Can it be delivered?
- **Film quality control:** How often is it necessary to repeat an exam? How many people are involved in quality control? Who is responsible for it?
- **Complication rates:** Do they meet the rates reported in the literature? Can they be improved?
- **Observer variability:** Variability between interpretations provided by different radiologists must diminish in order to promote the best interests of the customers (patients) as well as the radiologists. Ideally, a physician should be able to consult with anyone in the group and receive a reasonably similar differential diagnosis or workup recommendation.
- **Predictive values:** Determining the certainty of diagnosis is a most important factor to the referring physician. It is a function of specificity, sensitivity, and disease prevalence. All three can be controlled to some extent by (a) getting the most out of an exam, (b) integrating clinical knowledge of the patient, and (c) using clinically proven indicators for exams.
- **Expanding the focus:** In the spirit of the JCAHO's agenda for change, expand improvement beyond the walls of radiology in a spirit of cooperation with other departments in the hospital. Consider improving interdisciplinary care issues and how improved access/diagnosis will affect them.

Many opportunities for improvement in healthcare can be addressed directly by diagnostic radiology, even though the overall responsibilities cross departmental boundaries. Recall that one of Dr. Deming's points is to break down the barriers between departments and work together to solve problems and improve the services provided (point #9).

As outlined in the preceding chapters, TQM provides the framework for studying long known problems in the diagnosis and treatment of disease with the intent of improvement. As healthcare professionals undertaking the responsibility of healing, we all strive to do what is right for our patients. An integral part of doing what is right is seeking improvement in what we do today, to contribute to our profession and to contribute to the improvement of healthcare of tomorrow.

Examples of areas for improvement which cross artificial boundaries include:

- **Perforated appendices found at operation:** In the past, the surgeon was held responsible for interpreting this statistic. Can radiologists help improve this statistic? Can diagnostic criteria be improved to allow for earlier detection of appendicitis by improved sensitivity of ultrasound diagnosis, some other examination, or a combination thereof?
- **Normal appendectomy rate:** Once again, this is a surgical problem, but can radiologists as diagnosticians help to improve this rate? Can ultrasound diagnosis of the abdomen improve the false-positive rate of appendectomy?
- **Ruptured ectopic rate:** This morbidity statistic is usually the responsibility of the OB/GYN. Can radiologists improve this rate by improving the service provided in diagnosis?
- **Post-traumatic spleen salvage rate:** Following splenic injury, are there diagnostic clues that favor watching the patient instead of removing the injured organ?

These are cross-functional responsibilities where the efforts of the radiologists can enhance the utility of diagnostic radiology to other physicians, as well as benefit patients.

Overall, a decrease in the cost of care may be achieved by identifying high yield diagnostic pathways, improving or minimizing the use of low yield examinations that have little influence on patient outcome, providing earlier and more certain diagnosis through the use of innovative diagnostic science, and by decreasing complications. For example, must all data be reported in a binary format (positive/negative)?

Can diagnostic schemes be developed for high-cost imaging technologies, similar to scintigraphic diagnosis of pulmonary embolism? To do so, such examinations must be evaluated in terms of high positive and negative predictive values. If the predictive value is high enough, no further workup may be needed. However, in the indeterminate category, further workup may be needed to improve diagnostic certainty.

Figure 9.14 is an adaptation of Figure 6.5 in which the results table is refined to include an area where overlap of the diseased and non-diseased populations makes prediction of the presence of disease problematic. Using this type of analysis can potentially improve positive and negative predictive values, reduce the cost and time of diagnostic workups, and provide better care. The example of the diagnostic workup of PE illustrates this point. It was designed to demonstrate a better way to diagnose the presence or absence of this disease.

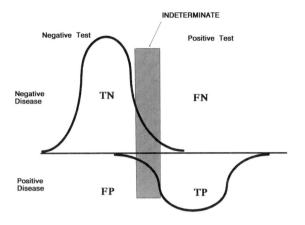

Figure 9.14 Modified Results Table

The graph in Figure 9.14 represents a disease and non-disease population. The area of overlap indicates where there is poor predictive value for a given exam. Patients whose exams places them in this region should theoretically be referred for more specific examinations. The workups of those patients at the extremes, with high positive or negative predictive values, could theoretically be ended at this point, thus eliminating the time and expense of additional exams.

10

The USE of PERSONAL COMPUTERS in the IMPROVEMENT PROCESS

The ease with which humans employ computer systems depends on three related factors: (1) the skill and experience of the user, (2) the importance to the user of a solution to a particular problem, and (3) the human engineering that went into the development of the system.

Marsden S. Blois
Information and Medicine
University of California Press, 1984

It is apparent from the examples in the previous chapters that a great amount of data drives the improvement process. Data processing, therefore, is essential in assisting the improvement effort. This data processing does not require highly sophisticated programmers or a detailed knowledge of computers. It does require a knowledge of what data must be obtained and what to do with it.

This section assumes that the reader had some knowledge of computers and current software programs. It is not intended to be an extensive tutorial on the use of personal computers or software packages.

Many reliable computer systems are currently available for around $1000.00 that will run current database and spreadsheet software. This should include at a minimum a dot matrix printer and a black and white video display monitor.

DATA COLLECTION AND ENTRY

This is probably the most important step in the information process. In order to have the least impact on the operation, data collection and entry should be made an integral part of the department routine. Capturing small pieces of information as a normal part of the daily routine has little or no impact.

For example, in the patient waiting time project, the time slips were attached to a random sample of radiographic requests and entered into the database at the end of each day. If a radiology information system is in place, it may be possible to capture certain pieces of information using the existing system or it may be possible to modify the system to act as a database.

In the report turnaround project, the radiologists were instructed in how to provide the information needed as an essential part of the reporting process (i.e., dates and times of exams and dictations were included in the dictations and transcribed in the reports). Reports were sampled, and data were entered on a regular basis. Allowing the data entry to pile up made it more difficult to tackle.

Gathering information is not much different in clinical improvement projects. Capturing necessary information at the time of the examination is much more efficient than gathering the information by reviewing records at a later date. Once again, the assistance of a statistician will likely save time and improve the quality of the information obtained.

DATABASES

Relational databases are computer programs that allow the user to organize pieces of information into specific categories, similar to an address book that contains names, addresses, cities, states, zip codes, and phone numbers. The database program organizes the data into tables (Figure 10.1); the data can be retrieved or processed to yield statistical information about the "population" of data entries contained in the database.

Each column in a database is called a *field* and each row a *record*. The intersection of a column and a row is a *field entry*.

Databases that have statistical functions are the most efficacious for the improvement process. Stand-alone, user-friendly programs can be created that allow non-computer-literate people to enter the data.

The design of the database is of critical importance. There must be some sense of what information is needed in order to obtain usable

```
            FIELD 1      FIELD 2      FIELD 3      FIELD 4    .  .  .      FIELD N
RECORD 1    .......      .......      .......      .......                 .......
RECORD 2    .......      .......      .......      .......                 .......
RECORD 3    .......      .......      .......      .......                 .......
   .
   .
   .
RECORD M    .......      .......      .......      .......                 .......
```

Figure 10.1A Architecture of a Relational Database

```
            NAME       ADDRESS        CITY       STATE     ZIP       PHONE
RECORD 1    JOHN DOE   12 5TH AVE     NEW YORK   NY        00131     (926) 555-1212
RECORD 2    JANE DOAN  66 SUNSET ST   BEVERLY    CA        90210     (714) 999-0000
RECORD 3    .....
   .
   .
   .
RECORD X    .....      ETC.
```

Figure 10.1B Example of Address Database

information. It may be preferable to identify the desired results first and then define the information that must be captured in order to obtain those results.

Using the patient waiting time project as an example, look at the original database designed. It was (1) designed to provide the total time the patient waited in the department for a finished product and (2) broken into logical time segments that would help focus attention on areas of possible delay. Thus, fields were defined for the times that were recorded and the patient and exam information; these fields would be used to sort or filter the information (Figure 10.2).

For example, there was a need to determine whether or not the departmental policy of giving priority to emergency room patients resulted in decreased waiting time. Thus, a method was needed to identify those patients so that they could be separated from the other patients and their waiting time averages computed separately.

Different exam types were also selected because this particular facility had dedicated chest rooms for which it was hypothesized that the waiting time should be less. Recall that one of the basic tenets of TQM is that hypotheses are tested using data. As above, the need to select different exam types required that a field for exam type be defined.

The astute reader will notice that the original database contained fields defined for each of the different exam and patient types, with an "x" entered in the field if the patient met the definition of the type. A more efficient database would have a field defined only for patient type

DATE	CHEST	OUTPT	ER	INPATIENT	URG	CHECKIN	ROOM	COMPLETE	READING	CHK-RM	RM-CMPLT	READ	T_WAIT
05/01/90	X				X	0940	0955	1006		15	11	#VALUE!	26
05/01/90	X				X	0904	0930	0938		26	8	#VALUE!	34
05/01/90		X	X			0930	0957	1002		27	5	#VALUE!	32
05/03/90		X				0904	0908	0921		4	13	#VALUE!	17
05/03/90		X			X	1025	1110	1125		45	15	#VALUE!	60
05/03/90		X			X	1202	1218	1234		16	16	#VALUE!	32
05/04/90	X			X		1100	1132	1220	1500	32	48	160	240
05/04/90	X				X	1317	1321	1329		4	8	#VALUE!	12
05/04/90			X			1305	1325	1333		20	8	#VALUE!	28
05/04/90	X		X			1200	1210	1221		10	11	#VALUE!	21
05/04/90	X				X	1136	1150	1155	1200	14	5	5	24
05/04/90	X				X	1145	1155	1159	1201	10	4	2	16
05/04/90	X				X	1115	1125	1130	1207	10	5	37	52
05/04/90					X	1121	1135	1141		14	6	#VALUE!	20
05/04/90	X		X			1012	1024	1040	1053	12	16	13	41
05/04/90	X		X			1017	1030	1040	1055	13	10	15	38
05/04/90					X	1016	1025	1040		9	15	#VALUE!	24
05/04/90	X				X	0950	1000	1024	1053	10	24	29	63
05/04/90	X				X	0928	0942	0954	1000	14	12	6	32
05/04/90	X				X	0901	0915	0935	0955	14	20	20	54

DATE	EXTYPE	PTTYPE	CHECKIN	ROOM	COMPLETE	READING	CHK-RM	RM-CMPLT	READ	T_WAIT
05/01/90	CXR	URG	0940	0955	1006		15	11	#VALUE!	26
05/01/90	CXR	URG	0904	0930	0938		26	8	#VALUE!	34
05/01/90	ROUT	OPT	0930	0957	1002		27	5	#VALUE!	32
05/03/90	ROUT	ER	0904	0908	0921		4	13	#VALUE!	17
05/03/90	ROUT	URG	1025	1110	1125		45	15	#VALUE!	60
05/03/90	CXR	URG	1202	1218	1234		16	16	#VALUE!	32
05/04/90	CXR	INPT	1100	1132	1220	1500	32	48	160	240
05/04/90	CXR	URG	1317	1321	1329		4	8	#VALUE!	12
05/04/90	ROUT	ER	1305	1325	1333		20	8	#VALUE!	28
05/04/90	CXR	URG	1200	1210	1221		10	11	#VALUE!	21
05/04/90	CXR	URG	1136	1150	1155	1200	14	5	5	24
05/04/90	CXR	URG	1145	1155	1159	1201	10	4	2	16

Figure 10.2 Improvement in Database Design by Consolidating Patient and Exam Type

and a code for type entered in the field, thus eliminating the need for three of the five fields used to identify patient and exam type.

Time fields were defined to contain the times recorded on the time slips. This was all that was needed for data entry. The project was designed so that the computer would do as much work as possible; therefore, calculated fields were added to show the time intervals between the entered times. Averages and standard deviations were derived from these calculated fields.

The reader will also notice that there are error messages in the calculated field READTIME (#VALUE!). This indicates that there was no entry for the reading of the exam. The exam was not classified as a "wet read" and therefore did not contribute to patient waiting time. This "error" is used by the database to filter out the "wet reads" and calculate these averages and standard deviations instead of adding an additional field for "wet reads." This is effective if the error can be trapped and total time calculated irrespective of the error.

The computer was also programmed to calculate waiting time averages and standard deviations for sampled patients distributed by the time of day the patients arrived in the department. In other words, the data were sequentially sorted by time of arrival, and waiting times were averaged for each subgroup.

Counts were added to evaluate the validity of the data calculated. A smaller data set or number of patients sampled in each subgroup yielded less reliable data. A patient identity number was added later in the improvement process to allow identification of any patient that exceeded the upper control limit for waiting time. This allowed the improvement team to determine why the patient waited so long and what could be done to keep this from occurring again.

For larger databases, it is recommended that the data be grouped logically and separate database files be created and *linked* by certain index fields. For example, using the index field patient ID number, one database could contain patient demographic information (name, address, phone, etc.), and a second database could contain exam information and results. Each file would contain the patient ID field in addition to the other information required. Each file would be linked by the patient ID index field (Figure 10.3).

Another sample database was used to evaluate report turnaround time. This particular facility wanted to study the turnaround times for its ICU/CCU patients, other inpatients (IP), emergency room (ER) patients, and outpatients (OP). The raw data in the database and the layout are provided in Figure 10.4. It begins with a computer-generated record number that allows the database to be audited (see later) for validity. It

Database #1

PATIENT DEMOGRAPHICS

	(INDEX) PT ID #	PT NAME	ADDR	CITY	. . .	ECT
RECORD 1	1111111	PT 1	....	....		....
RECORD 2	2222222	PT 2...	....	....		....
RECORD 3	3333333	....	....	....		....
.						
.						
.						
RECORD M	MMMMMM	....	....	....		....

Database #2

EXAM INFORMATION

	(INDEX) PT ID #	EXAMDATE	EXAMTYPE	RADIOL	TECH	INTERP	PEEREV
RECORD 1	1111111	10/30/92	MAMMO	NYD	APB	B9	MALIG
RECORD 2	1111111	12/13/92	BONE SCAN	ABC	NM	POS	NEG
RECORD 3	2222222	02/15/93	CXR	DEF	CM	NEG	NEG
.							
.							
RECORD X	.....	ETC.					

Figure 10.3 Example of Databases Linked by an Index Field

then houses information about the randomly sampled reports from which date and time of exam, dictation, transcription, and delivery were obtained.

The data was processed in a printed report format (Figure 10.5) which added calculated fields for the time intervals from exam to dictation, dictation to transcription, and transcription to delivery and the total turnaround time from exam to report on the chart. The processed report also contained calculated fields capable of generating the means and standard deviations for the population set consisting of all patients and the subsets ER, ICU/CCU, IP, and OP.

Why not just print the time intervals and the total times rather than include the raw data as well? It is preferable to print all the data until confident in the accuracy of the data entry and the computations performed by the software. Printing the raw data also provides a quick audit of the data in case one or more of the computed values is unexpected.

REC NO.	REQ LOC	EXAM DATE	EXAM TIME	DICT DATE	DICT TIME	TRANSC DATE	TRANSC TIME	DELIV DATE	DELIV TIME
1	OP	19930224	1436	19930225	1516	19930226	950	19930226	1405
2	ICU	19930225	800	19930225	1641	19930226	1000	19930226	1410
3	IP	19930225	1137	19930225	1528	19930226	954	19930226	1406
4	ICU	19930223	1840	19930224	923	19930224	1109	19930225	815
5	ER	19930224	1400	19930224	2017	19930225	1038	19930225	1300
6	ER	19930223	2150	19930224	850	19930224	1038	19930225	945
7	IP	19930223	829	19930223	1616	19930224	856	19930224	1500
8	IP	19930224	939	19930224	2014	19930225	1053	19930225	1315
9	IP	19930225	1120	19930225	1524	19930226	953	19930226	1405
10	IP	19930222	1457	19930223	1600	19930224	1159	19930224	1530
11	ICU	19930314	1520	19930315	818	19930315	1018	19930315	1115
12	ICU	19930228	2400	19930301	1023	19930302	944	19930302	1435
13	ICU	19930303	1640	19930304	740	19930304	1340	19930304	1400
14	ICU	19930308	1410	19930308	2035	19930309	1644	19930310	800
15	ICU	19930310	1615	19930310	1920	19930311	1501	19930311	2222
16	IP	19930301	630	19930301	1415	19930302	1011	19930302	1435
17	IP	19930302	1150	19930302	1950	19930303	1605	19930303	1900
18	IP	19930308	2350	19930309	840	19930309	1630	19930309	2200
19	IP	19930309	2110	19930310	810	19930310	1648	19930310	2200

Figure 10.4 Database Layout for Report Turnaround Time

05/10/93

RECNO	REQLOC	EXDATE	EXTIME	TIME1	DICDATE	DICTIME	TIME2	TRANSDATE	TRANSTIME	TIME3	DELIVDATE	DELIVTIME	TOTIME
1	OP	02/24/93	1436	24.80	02/25/93	1516	18.34	02/26/93	950	4.55	02/26/93	1405	47.69 Hours
2	ICU	02/25/93	800	8.41	02/25/93	1641	17.59	02/26/93	1000	4.10	02/26/93	1410	30.10 Hours
3	IP	02/25/93	1137	3.91	02/25/93	1528	18.26	02/26/93	954	4.52	02/26/93	1406	26.69 Hours
4	ICU	02/23/93	1840	14.83	02/24/93	923	1.86	02/24/93	1109	21.06	02/25/93	815	37.75 Hours
5	ER	02/24/93	1400	6.17	02/24/93	2017	14.21	02/25/93	1038	2.62	02/25/93	1300	23.00 Hours
6	ER	02/23/93	2150	11.00	02/24/93	850	1.88	02/24/93	1038	23.07	02/25/93	945	35.95 Hours
7	IP	02/23/93	829	7.87	02/23/93	1616	16.40	02/24/93	856	6.44	02/24/93	1500	30.71 Hours
8	IP	02/24/93	939	10.75	02/24/93	2014	14.39	02/25/93	1053	2.62	02/25/93	1315	27.76 Hours
9	IP	02/25/93	1120	4.04	02/25/93	1524	18.29	02/26/93	953	4.52	02/26/93	1405	26.85 Hours
10	IP	02/22/93	1457	25.43	02/23/93	1600	19.59	02/24/93	1159	3.71	02/24/93	1530	48.73 Hours
11	ICU	03/14/93	1520	16.98	03/15/93	818	2.00	03/15/93	1018	0.97	03/15/93	1115	19.95 Hours
12	ICU	02/28/93	2400	10.23	03/01/93	1023	23.21	03/02/93	944	4.91	03/02/93	1435	38.35 Hours
13	ICU	03/03/93	1640	15.00	03/04/93	740	6.00	03/04/93	1340	0.60	03/04/93	1400	21.60 Hours
14	ICU	03/08/93	1410	6.25	03/08/93	2035	20.09	03/09/93	1644	15.56	03/10/93	800	41.90 Hours
15	ICU	03/10/93	1615	3.05	03/10/93	1920	19.81	03/11/93	1501	7.21	03/11/93	2222	30.07 Hours
16	IP	03/01/93	630	7.85	03/01/93	1415	19.96	03/02/93	1011	4.24	03/02/93	1435	32.05 Hours
17	IP	03/02/93	1150	8.00	03/02/93	1950	20.55	03/03/93	1605	2.95	03/03/93	1900	31.50 Hours
18	IP	03/08/93	2350	8.90	03/09/93	840	7.90	03/09/93	1630	5.70	03/09/93	2200	22.50 Hours
19	IP	03/09/93	2110	11.00	03/10/93	810	8.38	03/10/93	1648	5.52	03/10/93	2200	24.90 Hours

. . . . .

AVE DICTATION TIME:	7.01	AVE TRANS TIME:	7.59	AVE DELIV TIME:	6.96	AVE TURN AROUND TIME:	21.56 HOURS
STANDARD DEVIATION:	7.62		8.84		7.77		15.99

Figure 10.5 Report Turnaround Time Computed as a Database Report

	A	B	C	D	E	F	G	H	I	J	K
1	0	0	0	0	0	0	0	0	0	0	0
2	0	0	0	0	0	0	0	0	0	0	0
3	0	0	0	0	0	0	0	0	0	0	0
4	0	0	0	0	0	0	0	0	0	0	0
5	0	0	0	0	0	0	0	0	0	0	0
6	0	0	0	0	0	0	0	0	0	0	0
7	0	0	0	0	0	0	0	0	0	0	0
8	0	0	0	0	0	0	0	0	0	0	0
9	0	0	0	0	0	0	0	0	0	0	0
10	0	0	0	0	0	0	0	0	0	0	0
11	0	0	0	0	0	0	0	0	0	0	0
12	0	0	0	0	0	0	0	0	0	0	0
13	0	0	0	0	0	0	0	0	0	0	0
14	0	0	0	0	0	0	0	0	0	0	0
15	0	0	0	0	0	0	0	0	0	0	0
16	0	0	0	0	0	0	0	0	0	0	0
17	0	0	0	0	0	0	0	0	0	0	0
18	0	0	0	0	0	0	0	0	0	0	0
19	0	0	0	0	0	0	0	0	0	0	0
20	0	0	0	0	0	0	0	0	0	0	0
21	0	0	0	0	0	0	0	0	0	0	0
22	0	0	0	0	0	0	0	0	0	0	0
23	0	0	0	0	0	0	0	0	0	0	0
24	0	0	0	0	0	0	0	0	0	0	0
25	0	0	0	0	0	0	0	0	0	0	0
26	0	0	0	0	0	0	0	0	0	0	0
27	0	0	0	0	0	0	0	0	0	0	0
28	0	0	0	0	0	0	0	0	0	0	0
29	0	0	0	0	0	0	0	0	0	0	0
30	0	0	0	0	0	0	0	0	0	0	0
31	0	0	0	0	0	0	0	0	0	0	0
32	0	0	0	0	0	0	0	0	0	0	0
33	0	0	0	0	0	0	0	0	0	0	0
34	0	0	0	0	0	0	0	0	0	0	0
35	0	0	0	0	0	0	0	0	0	0	0

Figure 10.6 Spreadsheet

SPREADSHEETS

A spreadsheet is a rectangular grid of columns and rows into which data can be entered to produce useful information. The basic unit of a spreadsheet is a *cell,* which is the intersection of a column and a row in which data are stored. Columns are labeled from left to right (usually with letters). Rows are usually numbered from top to bottom through the extent of the worksheet (Figure 10.6). A spreadsheet is filled in by entering text, numbers, or formulas in the cells.

The way information is displayed in the worksheet can be altered by changing the size, style, and color of data within the cells. Most software allows graphic objects to be added to enhance the appearance of the worksheet.

Some programs allow multiple spreadsheets to be linked. For example, several spreadsheets that calculate monthly financial data can be linked to calculate quarterly data. When spreadsheets are linked, changes made in one spreadsheet result in corresponding changes in the linked spreadsheets.

The difference between a database and a spreadsheet is that the individual cells in a spreadsheet can be easily referenced and redefined to provide any format desired. The columns in a database are fixed as defined and cannot be otherwise defined without redefining the entire column.

While most current spreadsheet programs have many of the same functions as database programs, a preference for databases stems primarily from the ease of data entry. There does not appear to be any easy way to modify the entry screen for a spreadsheet to look like the data collection form that was used. Using a computer screen that looks like the data sheet is less likely to produce data entry errors than entering information in a monotonous grid such as a spreadsheet screen.

A spreadsheet, however, can be used as a tool to produce formatted reports of results from a database if the spreadsheet is compatible with and can read the database file.

For example, the patient waiting time data derived from a database was displayed on a spreadsheet. The spreadsheet was programmed to process the database information and produce information relevant to the improvement project. As illustrated in Figure 10.7, information was derived for different patient types, different exam types, and different times of day and displayed in a readable format.

Each data cell was programmed to provide the information displayed. For example, cell B4 contains a hidden program that accesses the database containing patient waiting times, filters the database for patients whose exams were requested as "wet reads," and computes and displays the average waiting times from check-in to exam room. The average waiting time from room time to exam completed is calculated and displayed in cell C4, and the average waiting time for a reading is calculated and displayed in cell D4. The average total waiting time is calculated and displayed in cell E4, and the total number of patients counted in this filtered database is displayed in cell F4. Three times the standard deviation is calculated and displayed in cell G4, the maximum waiting time for the filtered database is found in cell H4, and the minimum waiting time is found in cell I4.

Cell J4 is a check to be used in evaluating the significance of the total waiting times. In the filtered database showing only "wet reads," this cell should equal cell F4, which it does. All ER patients should be "wet reads" as per the policy of the facility, and therefore cell J8 should equal cell F8.

When looking at the breakdown by time of day, the number of "wet reads" can serve to show the validity of the reading time averages. Sample sizes with low numbers will yield results that should not be considered representative of the actual reading time.

	A	B	C	D	E	F	G	H	I	J
		CKIN-RM	RM-CMPLT	READ	TOTAL	NUM PTS	3STDEV	MAX	MIN	NUM READS
1										
2										
3										
4	WET READS	16.33	14.60	24.07	55.00	43	86	160.00	25.00	43
5	NON WETS	21.85	11.18	N/A	33.03	78	56	125.00	9.00	0
6	INPTS	18.09	9.73	N/A	27.82	11	48	60.00	9.00	0
7	ADINUNIF	17.33	11.97	11.75	32.43	30	71	137.00	10.00	8
8	ER PTS	11.00	13.00	19.43	43.43	7	44	76.00	33.00	7
9	OTHERS	22.05	12.92	28.75	46.00	73	78	160.00	15.00	28
10	CHEST	20.64	9.80	26.70	36.87	83	72	160.00	9.00	20
11	OTHER EX	18.38	17.48	21.67	48.24	42	73	137.00	20.00	24
12	OVERALL	19.88	12.40	24.07	40.83	121	75	160.00	9.00	43
13										
14	0700-0800	16.00	24.67	5.00	42.33	3	58	55.00	20.00	1
15	0800-0900	12.50	11.71	40.57	44.50	14	111	160.00	9.00	7
16	0900-1000	19.54	10.20	20.91	36.31	35	63	105.00	10.00	11
17	1000-1100	24.45	13.45	21.29	45.74	38	81	137.00	15.00	14
18	1100-1200	15.67	11.33	31.40	40.08	12	67	82.00	15.00	5
19	1200-1300	17.86	15.14	12.50	36.57	7	74	88.00	15.00	2
20	1300-1400	12.00	11.67	8.00	26.33	3	7	29.00	25.00	1
21	1400-1500	29.83	14.33	9.00	45.67	6	58	76.00	23.00	1
22	1500-1600	18.50	10.50	19.00	38.50	2	6	40.00	37.00	1
23										
24	MAX	29.83	24.67	40.57	55.00					
25	MIN	11.00	9.73	5.00	26.33					
26										
27				% WET READS	35.54					
28										

Figure 10.7 Spreadsheet Display of the Patient Waiting Time Database

AUDITS

The computer axiom *garbage in, garbage out* means that the information retrieved is only as good as the data from which it is derived. This emphasizes the need to audit the database to improve the validity of the information.

There are a number of ways this can be accomplished. One way is to print out the database whenever data entry is completed and review the calculated fields as well as the data entered to determine whether any values appear to be erroneous. For example, a time interval with a negative number indicates a mistake.

Another way is to program a *check* into the data entry program. In the report turnaround time program, a table was created from which a REQUESTING LOCATION can be entered by simply pressing a key, thus reducing the likelihood of error. Individual fields can be programmed to accept only certain types of entries, and calculated fields can be programmed to give a message to the person doing the data entry if the calculation indicates the possibility of an erroneous entry.

The number of samples is another way to determine the validity of the data. A small sample size will not carry much statistical significance. A good example of this is the patient waiting time project. The data in Figure 10.8 show an increased overall waiting time of 67 minutes. A quick look at the percentage of "wet reads" identifies a significant contributing factor. Most of the patients sampled (87%) were "wet reads," which takes longer than those patients who do not wait for a reading. The "non-wet read" patients waited an average of 37 minutes.

The cause of this anomaly was the mistaken belief on the part of reception personnel that they were measuring only "wet read" patients. Plan, Do, Check, Act.

Another audit alluded to earlier can be conducted by assigning record numbers to the data entered. For example, the reports that were randomly sampled could be easily retrieved if an entry error yielded a calculation that did not fit the expected result. In fact, this is an excellent improvement tool in that those reports that fall outside the limit of three standard deviations can be examined and researched to determine the special cause of the extremely high or low turnaround time. Any report that exceeds +3 standard deviations indicates a breakdown in the system and will yield important improvement information. Any report that exceeds the limit of −3 standard deviations potentially holds the key to a breakthrough in improvement.

	CKIN-RM	RM-CMPLT	READ	TOTAL	NUM PTS	3STDEV	MAX	MIN	NUM READS
WET READS	16.24	17.29	38.22	71.75	**173**	125	240.00	18.00	173
NON WETS	16.15	20.88	N/A	37.04	26	60	78.00	10.00	0
INPTS	17.75	17.88	76.00	83.13	8	191	222.00	20.00	5
ADINUNIF	15.17	15.61	40.93	68.24	59	116	170.00	10.00	54
ER PTS	23.00	16.22	16.67	55.89	9	61	85.00	30.00	9
OTHERS	16.14	18.89	36.88	66.51	123	125	240.00	10.00	105
CHEST	17.05	15.38	43.02	69.56	117	141	240.00	10.00	101
OTHER EX	15.05	21.16	31.49	63.85	82	93	169.00	14.00	72
OVERALL	16.23	17.76	38.22	**67.21**	199	124	240.00	10.00	173
0700-0800	24.00	17.17	168.75	153.67	6	271	240.00	44.00	4
0800-0900	12.43	16.03	50.81	67.66	35	131	166.00	14.00	27
0900-1000	15.00	14.95	34.31	62.70	44	98	170.00	10.00	42
1000-1100	18.47	18.70	34.53	68.77	47	119	240.00	15.00	43
1100-1200	16.72	23.52	33.65	66.93	29	107	169.00	25.00	23
1200-1300	12.60	17.67	24.38	51.40	15	61	85.00	20.00	13
1300-1400	20.00	13.00	31.09	64.09	11	91	130.00	20.00	11
1400-1500	19.75	26.38	22.63	68.75	8	77	111.00	35.00	8
1500-1600	17.50	8.00	12.50	31.75	4	52	52.00	10.00	2
MAX	24.00	26.38	168.75	153.67					
MIN	12.43	8.00	12.50	31.75					

% WET READS **86.93**

Figure 10.8 Monthly Display Showing a High Number of Wet Reads and an Increased Overall Waiting Time as a Result

HARDWARE REQUIREMENTS

Adequate storage capacity in the computer system is important in order to avoid frustrating hours of re-entering data lost when the capacity of the system is unexpectedly reached. The simplest way to compute system storage requirements is to add up the characters allotted for each field in a record. Multiply this by the number of records expected over the time frame of the study. This will give an approximation of how much memory storage area (hard or floppy disk capacity) will be needed (Figure 10.9).

Database File

```
           FIELD 1   FIELD 2   FIELD 3   FIELD 4    .   .   .   FIELD N
RECORD 1   .......   .......   .......   .......                .......
RECORD 2   .......   .......   .......   .......                .......
RECORD 3   .......   .......   .......   .......                .......
.
.
RECORD M   .......   .......   .......   .......                .......
```

Approximate mass storage requirements = #expected records X (#characters Field 1 +
                                        #characters Field 2 + . . . #characters Field N)

Example Database File

```
           NAME        ADDRESS       CITY       STATE    ZIP       PHONE
RECORD 1   JOHN DOE    12 5TH AVE    NEW YORK   NY       00131     (926) 555-1212
RECORD 2   JANE DOAN   66 SUNSET ST  BEVERLY    CA       90210     (714) 999-0000
RECORD 3   .....
.          [   -9-  ] [    -14-    ] [  -9-  ] [ 2 ]    [ -7- ]   [    -13-    ]
.
RECORD 100 ....        ETC.
```

Approximate mass storage requirements = 100 X (9 + 14 + 9 + 2 + 7 + 13)

                                      = 5400 Bytes (5.4 Kbytes)

Figure 10.9 Calculation of Disk Storage Requirements

Appendix A

QUALITY IMPROVEMENT TEMPLATES

Template #1

PROCESS WORKSHEET

Process Worksheet: Define the Basic Processes in the Flowchart						
Proc#	Supplier	Input	Action	Output	Customer	Needs & Expectations

Template #2

DATA COLLECTION WORKSHEET

Process:

Owner:

Current Actions:

Needs/Expectations (Key Quality Characteristics):

Sources of Variation (Key Process Variables):

Data Needed:

How Data to be Acquired:

When Data is Required:

Template #3

RADIOLOGY TIME SLIP

Exam Date:

    Times:

        Arrival [_____]

        Room [_____]

        Complete [_____]

        Dismissed [_____]

Exam Type:

[ ]   Chest

[ ]   Other

[ ]   Wet Read

PT Type:

[ ]   OP

[ ]   IP

[ ]   ER

[ ]   URG

Template #4

CONTINUOUS IMPROVEMENT ACTION WORKSHEET

Problem:

Current Solution:

Plan: Goals:

                   Methods:

Do: Training:

                   Implementation Target:

Check:

Act:

ADDITIONAL READINGS

Chapter 1

1. Dentzer S: How to fight killer healthcare costs. *US News and World Report* September 23, 1991, pp 50–58.
2. Deming WE: *Out of the Crisis,* Cambridge, Mass.: MIT Press, 1986.
3. Walton M: *The Deming Management Method,* Perigee Press, 1989.
4. Drucker PF: *The Effective Executive,* New York: Harper & Row, 1967.
5. Peters TJ, Waterman RH: *In Search of Excellence,* New York: Harper & Row, 1982.
6. McLelland R, Hendrick RE, Zinninger MD, Wilcox PA: The American College of Radiology Mammography Accreditation Program, *AJR* 157:473–479, September 1991.
7. Kritchevesky SB, Simmons BP: Continuous quality improvement. *JAMA* 266:1817–1823, 1991.
8. Chassin MR: Quality of care: A time to act. *JAMA* 266:3472–3473, 1991.
9. Berwick DM: Continuous improvement as an ideal in health care. *NEJM* 320(1):53–56, January 5, 1989.
10. Relman AS: Assessment and accountability: The third revolution in medical care. *NEJM* 319:1220–1222, 1988.
11. Cascade P: Quality improvement in diagnostic radiology. *AJR* 154:1117–1120, May 1990.

Chapter 2

1. Deming WE: *Out of the Crisis,* Cambridge, Mass.: MIT Press, 1986.
2. Peters TJ, Austin N: *A Passion for Excellence: The Leadership Difference,* New York: Random House, 1985.
3. Peters TJ, Waterman RH: *In Search of Excellence,* New York: Harper & Row, 1982.
4. Crosby PB: *Quality Is Free: The Art of Making Quality Certain,* New York: McGraw-Hill, 1979.
5. Peters TJ: *Thriving on Chaos,* New York: Alfred A. Knopf, 1987.

Chapter 3

1. Ishikawa K: *What Is Total Quality Control? The Japanese Way,* Lu DJ (trans), Englewood Cliffs, N.J.: Prentice-Hall, 1985.
2. Deming WE: *Out of the Crisis,* Cambridge, Mass.: MIT Press, 1986.
3. *Accreditation Manual for Hospitals—Diagnostic Radiology,* Chicago: JCAHO, 1992.
4. McNeil BJ, Abrams HL (eds): *Brigham and Women's Hospital Handbook of Diagnostic Imaging,* Boston: Little, Brown, 1986.
5. Bulmer MG: *Principles of Statistics,* New York: Dover Publications, 1979.
6. Walton M: *Deming Management at Work,* New York: Putnam, 1990.

Chapter 4

1. Deming WE: *Out of the Crisis,* Cambridge, Mass.: MIT Press, 1986.
2. Walton M: *Deming Management at Work,* New York: Putnam, 1990.
3. Batalden P, Gillem T: *Hospitalwide Quality Improvement Storytelling,* Nashville: Hospital Corporation of America, 1989.
4. Scholtes PR: *The Team Handbook: How to Improve Quality With Teams,* Madison, Wisc.: Joiner Associates, 1988.

Chapter 5

1. Walton M: *Deming Management at Work,* New York: Putnam, 1990.
2. Ishikawa K: *What Is Total Quality Control? The Japanese Way,* Lu DJ (trans), Englewood Cliffs, N.J.: Prentice-Hall, 1985.

Chapter 6

1. Metz CE, ROC methodology in radiologic imaging. *Invest Radiol* 21:720–733, 1986.
2. Metz CE, Goodenough DJ, Rossmann K: Evaluation of ROC curve data in terms of information theory, with applications in radiology. *Rad* 109:297–303, November 1973.
3. McNeil BJ, Keeler E, Adelstein SJ: Primer on certain elements of medical decision making. *NEJM* 293:211–215, 1975.
4. Hanley JA: Alternative approaches to ROC analyses. *Rad* 168:568–570, 1988.
5. Black WC, Armstrong P: Communicating the significance of radiologic test results: The likelihood ratio. *AJR* 147:1313–1318, December 1986.
6. Flanagin A, Lundberg GD: Clinical decision making: Promoting the jump from theory to practice. *JAMA* 263(2):279–280, January 1990.
7. Hoy RJ: Choosing and evaluating diagnostic examinations, in Straub WH (ed): *Manual of Diagnostic Imaging,* Boston: Little, Brown, 1989.
8. Phillips WC, Scott JA, Blasczcynski G: Statistics for diagnostic procedures. *AJR* 140:1265–1270, June 1983.
9. Phillips WC, Scott JA, Blasczcynski G: Statistics for diagnostic procedures. *AJR* 141:409–411, August 1983.
10. Browner WS, Newman TB: Are all significant *P* values created equal? *JAMA* 257:2459–2463, 1987.

11. Brismar J: Understanding ROC curves: A graphic approach. *AJR* 157:1119–1121, November 1991.

12. Lohr KN: Outcomes measurement: Concepts and questions. *Inquiry* 25:37–50, Spring 1988.

13. Schrieber MH: Wilson's law of diminishing returns. *AJR* 138:786–788, April 1982.

14. Kritchevsky SB, Simmons BP: Continuous quality improvement: Concepts and applications for physician care. *JAMA* 266:1817–1823, 1991.

15. Bronson JG: The uncertain quest for diagnostic certainty: The cost-benefit ratio. *Decisions in Imaging Economics.*

16. Hulley SB, Cummings SR: *Designing Clinical Research,* Baltimore: Williams & Wilkins, 1988.

Chapter 7

1. Scholtes PR: *The Team Handbook: How to Improve Quality With Teams,* Madison, Wisc.: Joiner Associates, 1988.

Chapter 8

1. *The Deming Route to Quality and Productivity: Road Maps and Roadblocks.*

2. Scherkenbach WW: *Deming's Road to Continual Improvement,* SPC Press, 1991.

3. Deming WE: *The New Economics For Industry, Government, and Education,* Cambridge, Mass.: MIT Center for Advanced Engineering Study, 1993.

Chapter 9

1. *The Measurment Mandate,* Oakbrook Terrace, Ill.: JCAHO, 1993.

2. Eddy DM: Screening for breast cancer. *Ann Int Med* 111:389–399, 1989.

3. Sickles EA: Quality assurance. *Radiol Clin North Am* January 1992, pp 265–275.

4. Eddy DM: Three battles to watch in the 1990s. *JAMA* 270(4):520–526, 1993.

5. Geehr EC, Pine J: *Increasing Physician Involvement in Quality Improvement Programs,* ACPE, 1992.

6. Blumenthal D: Total quality management and physicians' clinical decisions. *JAMA* 269(21):2775–2778

7. The PIOPED investigators: Value of the ventilation/perfusion scan in acute pulmonary embolism: Results of the Prospective Investigation of Pulmonary Embolism Diagnosis (PIOPED). *JAMA* 263:2753–2759, 1990.

Chapter 10

1. Blois MS: *Information and Medicine: The Nature of Medical Descriptions,* University of California Press, 1984.

2. Christensen WW, Stearns, EI: *Microcomputers In Health Care Management,* Aspen, 1984.

3. Sellars D: *Computerizing Your Medical Office,* Medec Books, 1983.

4. Covvey HD, McAlister NH: *Computers in the Practice of Medicine,* Reading, Mass.: Addison Wesley, 1980.

5. *Computer Applications in the Evaluation of Physician Competence,* Chicago: American Board of Medical Specialties, 1984.

INDEX